INSTITUTE OF MEDICINE

Controls on Health Care

Papers of the Conference on Regulation in the Health Industry
January 7-9, 1974

NATIONAL ACADEMY OF SCIENCES
WASHINGTON, D.C. 1975

The work upon which this publication is based was performed pursuant to contract HEW-OS-74-95 with the Department of Health, Education, and Welfare.

Library of Congress Cataloging In Publication Data

Conference on Regulation in the Health Industry, Washington, D.C., 1974.
Controls on health care.

At head of title: Institute of Medicine.
Includes bibliographical references.
1. Medical economics–United States–Congresses. 2. Medical care, Cost of–United States–Congresses. 3. Medical care–Law and legislation–United States–Congresses. I. Institute of Medicine. II. Title. [DNLM: 1. Delivery of health care–U.S. 2. Economics, Medical–U.S. 3. Health services–U.S. W84 AA1 C7c 1974]
RA410.53.C654 1974 344'.73'04 75-10566

ISBN 0-309-02330-0

Available from

Printing and Publishing Office, National Academy of Sciences
2101 Constitution Avenue, N.W., Washington, D.C. 20418

Printed in the United States of America

Preface

This volume contains the principal papers presented at the Conference on Regulation in the Health Industry, held in Washington, D.C., on January 7, 8, and 9, 1974, under the sponsorship of the Institute of Medicine, National Academy of Sciences.

The conference was organized in response to the increasing interest nationwide in proposals to expand governmental regulation of the health industry. More than 20 states had already enacted certification-of-need legislation to control new construction and expansion of hospitals and other health care facilities, and such legislation was under consideration in additional states. More comprehensive regulation, including the regulation of rates of payment for health care providers, was under consideration or had been adopted in a few states. The federal Cost of Living Council was engaged in regulating health care prices, and there was speculation that the practice might be continued beyond the termination of general price regulation. Medicare and Medicaid had been authorized, in reimbursing providers, to disapprove capital expenditures that state or local health planning agencies had determined unwarranted. In Congress and the executive branch of the federal government, proposals were being generated for federally sponsored regulation of the supply and distribution of health manpower and facilities and the regulation of payment rates.

These pushes toward greater regulation occurred in the context of widespread dissatisfaction with the performance of the health care industry. There was concern about the rate of increase in health care costs (especially rapid since the enactment of Medicare and Medicaid in 1965), and about the inability of some segments of the population to have effective access to health care services while others had an oversupply of health facilities and personnel. Underlying these concerns was the prospect of enactment of a program for national health insurance, lending urgency to the question of what regulatory techniques might be effective in controlling and improving the health care system.

Notwithstanding the interest in regulatory proposals, there had not been much discussion of their potential effects on the distribution and costs of health services or the productivity of health care providers. The Institute of Medicine sponsored the conference to foster a more detailed examination of the problems and prospects for further regulation in the health care field.

Scholars and experts in regulation were invited to prepare papers on a variety of topics related to existing and proposed regulatory mechanisms in the health field, as well as on the developments in other regulated industries. At the conference, presentations of the papers on each major topic were followed by comments of an expert panel, whose members were asked to conduct dialogues with the speaker and each other rather than prepare formal responses. All the conference participants then engaged in further discussion of the topic in small group seminars. The conference program organization had two objectives: to give participants an informal opportunity to share and consider their experiences in the area of health care regulation, and to provide to a larger audience this collection of the formal papers around which the participants organized their discussion.

Invited participants for the conference included some 150 high-level staff members of the executive and legislative branches of the federal government, individuals engaged in regulatory activities at the federal and state levels, individuals whose experience enabled them to reflect the interests and experience of health care providers and of third-party payers, and others including scholars and experts in regulation.

The conference was initiated by the Institute of Medicine's Committee on National Health Care Plans, chaired by Henry Riecken, Ph.D., professor of behavioral sciences, University of Pennsylvania School of Medicine. The program was organized under the direction of a planning subcommittee headed by Morton Miller, executive vice president and chief actuary, Equitable Life Assurance Society of the United States. Other members of the subcommittee were the late Robert Eilers, Ph.D., executive director, Leonard Davis Institute, University of Pennsylvania; Alain Enthoven, Ph.D., Eccles professor of public and private management, Graduate School of Business, Stanford University; William B. Schwartz, M.D., Endicott professor and chairman, Department of Medicine, Tufts University School of Medicine; and Alonzo S. Yerby, M.D., professor and head, Department of Health Services Administration, Harvard School of Public Health. These subcommittee members presided at conference plenary sessions and also served as moderators of the small group seminars, as did J. F. Volker, president of the University of Alabama, who was not a member of the subcommittee.

The Institute of Medicine wishes to express appreciation for the major financial support of the conference provided through a contract from the Department of Health, Education, and Welfare, and for the additional support provided by the Health Staff Seminar of George Washington University. Special thanks are also due the members of the discussion panels (listed separately with each topic) whose efforts contributed greatly to the value of the conference.

It is our hope that this collection of papers will contribute to a further thoughtful examination of the issues in health care regulation and will be helpful to policymakers as the nation moves toward final consideration of national health insurance.

RUTH S. HANFT
PAUL C. RETTIG
Project Directors
Institute of Medicine

Contents

I

An Introduction to Regulation

A considerable body of regulation already exists at various levels of the nation's health enterprise. In this introductory paper Robert M. Ball, former Commissioner of Social Security, draws on his first-hand knowledge of management of the Medicare program to outline the strengths and limitations of governmental action, to review the regulatory structure that has been assembled piecemeal around the health care industry, and to conjecture that effective governmental controls will be no more stringent than required to motivate action in the desired direction.

Discussants of Mr. Ball's paper at the conference were Lewis H. Butler, LL.B., adjunct professor of health policy, Health Policy Program, University of California School of Medicine, at San Francisco, and Gerald Garvey, professor of politics, Princeton University.

ROBERT M. BALL
Scholar in Residence, Institute of Medicine

Background of Regulation in Health Care

When those who have particular responsibility for the organization of personal health care services get together, agreement on goals is generally easy. Objectives include reducing the incidence of illness, preserving and enhancing conditions that lead to further gains for biomedical research, facilitating translation of medical knowledge into improved medical practice, providing access to high-quality medical care for all Americans regardless of geographical location or income, preventing unnecessary care, and doing what is necessary to control rising costs. That there is little guarantee of the quality of the services offered is among the concerns expressed. There is also concern about the patient's difficulty in making rational choices in the selection of services. And there is concern generally about the patient's ability to find his way into and through the system.

Most of this will usually be conceded. What is difficult is deciding the method, or methods, best suited to attaining the goals and responding to the concerns. Specifically, how much intervention in the health care system by government is called for? What interventions would be useful? What should be avoided?

We are not dealing with an abstract issue. Health care in the United States is at present a subject of considerable government attention. Government is a third-party buyer of medical services. It grants funds under a variety of conditions designed to influence the behavior of the recipient. Courts render decisions significantly affecting the health care system. Government is a direct regulator of who can do what, under what conditions, and increasingly of what price can be charged.

We are conscious not only of this present situation but also of what is being proposed. Organizations representing major provider groups in the health care field, the labor movement and other consumer groups, the health insurance industry, and a large number of senators and congressmen all have proposals that in one way or another would lead to greater government involvement in health care. Equally significant is that, at the state level, the traditional function of licensing and the more recent voluntary planning activity is developing into the direct control of facility and service expansion and cost regulation. And in some places these activities seem to be evolving into comprehensive regulation covering the availability and quality of services, health manpower training policy, and rate setting. This is the situation as we meet to discuss the subject of regulation.

My comments fall under three broad headings: (1) personal health care services—what and who is to be regulated; (2) the health care market—its characteristics and recent developments; and (3) government intervention.

PERSONAL HEALTH CARE SERVICES

Services and Other Determinants of Health

It is clear that the availability of even the best preventive, curative, and rehabilitative health services is only one—and certainly not the most important one—of the factors that determine the general level of health of an individual or a population. Mortality rates and morbidity rates are largely determined by heredity, by a variety of environmental factors, and by the way in which the individual handles himself within the environment. Traditional public health measures relating to water supply, food and milk supply, and epidemic-causing agents still make the big difference in mortality and morbidity rates, along with many other environmental factors that have gained more recent public notice—the quality of air, the control of noise, exposure to an accident-causing environment, the effectiveness of drug production controls, and the incidence of deliberate violence of man against man. Also, it is probable that personal performance in relation to weight control, exercise, recreation, reaction to stress, and attitudes toward self, sex, and society are of greater importance than health care in determining the general level of health.

The secondary role of health care services might lead one to conclude that we are making too much of a fuss about something that is not of overwhelming importance. It is very likely true that if we were to divert a significant portion of the money spent on health services to genetic and environmental improvement, we would be doing more to raise the general level of health than what we are now doing. It is also quite probable that if we provided the poor with an adequate income, as compared with providing them with health services, there would be greater payoffs in better health. We undoubtedly pay too little attention to the most important determinants of health and expect too much of personal health care. In reality, we do not have such stark choices to make. Personal health services may be overvalued, but they are nevertheless important. There is an immediacy to the need for such services that cannot be balanced against statistical probabilities. That immediacy makes the services indispensable to the individual, regardless of how small a share he may have in determining the health level of whole populations.

Health services are now generally perceived as being one of the necessities of life, and on the whole it is correct that they are so perceived. If balance is to be restored between personal health care services and other determinants of health, it will probably come as the result of putting more emphasis on factors of environment, heredity, and health habits rather than less emphasis on health care services.

The Range of Health Care Services

As we consider the regulation of health care services, it seems important to bear in mind that we are talking about a great range of activities, responsive to very different health needs and varying in the degree to which, in a given instance, the service may be objectively demonstrated to be medically required. We are, for example, talking about many medical and surgical procedures that are demonstrably lifesaving and health-restoring. In the treatment of most infectious diseases, in many situations for which surgical intervention is appropriate, and in a variety of other situations, physicians are fairly certain of the treatment and it usually works. But in many other cases the diagnosis may be unclear or the accepted procedures may offer little hope of causing significant improvement. As we talk about the regulation of health services, we need to be conscious not only of the great successes and scientific marvels of modern medicine but also of the gaps in medical knowledge. A very significant proportion of health personnel time is spent in relieving discomfort and giving reassurance in situations where specific therapy has little, if any, utility. We need to be aware of the fact that we have made it possible for much larger numbers of people to survive to old age, with a consequent increase in the incidence of chronic disease and just "aches and pains." And we have developed a great variety of specialized mental health services that are quite different in character from traditional physical medicine.

Therefore, as we talk about the kinds of service that are subject to regulation, we need to have in mind a range that extends from services that can be demonstrated to make an immediate and clear difference between life and death, or health and disability, to those that may give comfort without cure, or that imperceptibly shade from treatment of serious mental illness into a variety of personal and family counselling services. The concept of medical necessity is indeed elusive.

Health Institutions and Personnel

Regulation of health services is complicated not only by the range of services to be covered but also by the variety of institutions and people engaged in providing those services—the ones being regulated. There are more than 7,000 hospitals—including state, federal, municipal, and both voluntary and proprietary community institutions. While the majority are general acute-care hospitals, there are also mental hospitals, special hospitals for children, the chronically ill, the military, veterans, and for special diseases. There are over 20,000 nursing homes, ranging from those providing highly skilled services to those providing custodial care. There are some 325,000 active physicians, the majority of whom are in fee-for-service solo practice, but also including many who practice in fee-for-service groups and in various forms of prepayment plans. There are nearly 100,000 active dentists and three-quarters of a million professionally active nurses. Added to the major institutions and professional practitioners are a variety of service organizations, including neighborhood health centers, community mental health centers, family planning clinics, surgical centers, renal dialysis centers, and some 40,000 retail drugstores. There are over 400 titles of allied health personnel. The health industry is the third largest in the country, accounting for 7.7 percent of the gross national product and employing more than 4.5 million people.

There is a variety of programs designed to pay for health services in addition to the individual patient paying for services out of pocket. Federal, state, and local governments operate needs-tested programs for low-income people; the federal government has a national health service for veterans and the military; the states require workmen's compensation; private commercial insurance and Blue Cross and Blue Shield provide individual coverage and underwrite large-scale group plans; there is an increasing number of group practice prepayment plans; and the federal government operates a large-scale health insurance program for older people and the totally disabled.

My point in this recitation is simply a reminder of how varied are the services, institutions, and personnel to be regulated. This should not necessarily discourage us, but it does make the task extremely complicated.

THE HEALTH CARE MARKET

Attitudes Toward the Free Market and Regulation

The United States' attitude toward regulation of industry has been ambivalent. Most of us begin with concern that direct government regulation is likely to retard innovation, result in the protection of the status quo at the expense of the broad public interest, and restrict consumer choices. We have considerable faith in the idea that, since individual desires and wishes vary from one person to another, the best way to increase the sum total of human satisfaction is to let each individual select among a wide variety of possibilities. We tend to believe that out of this "democracy of the market place" there will be constant improvements in products as one producer tries to outdo another in attracting consumers on the basis of quality, price, and service. Consequently, we are inclined to turn toward regulation only when we are convinced that the scale required for the economic operation of an enterprise is such that monopoly is inevitable and that competition cannot be depended upon to keep prices at a reasonable level and service and quality acceptable.

Yet, as I have suggested, our attitude is ambivalent. Direct regulation is very appealing when matters do not seem to be going well. Regulation seems to be the approach that addresses itself most directly to the perceived problem. If prices are "too high," set rates; if desired services are not available in some area or for some people, fix the responsibility on some institution or organization to see that they are made available; if the quality of service is too low, set standards. Alternatives that involve incentives for performance seem indirect and do not have the appeal of an immediate solution, whereas goals and requirements can be written into law and into regulations giving the appearance, at least, of having solved the problem. We sometimes don't stop to realize that ordering a man to jump ten feet in the air doesn't make it possible for him to do so.

I am not raising the question of our attitudes toward the free market and regulation in order to pose an issue between the theoretical absolutes of a completely free health care market on the one hand, and completely detailed regulation of the industry on the other. Few people are going to quarrel with some type of minimal licensing designed to protect the public from the grossest forms of incompetence and fraud, and few people will quarrel with the desirability of better incentives for improved market performance. I am raising the question of our underlying attitudes to suggest that we may be right to be ambivalent—to want some of both. The realistic problem before the conference may well be the extent to which incentives can be improved *and* the extent to which direct regulation is useful.

Improving Market Functioning

The first category of activities to be considered here are those related to the improvement of the medical care market. There are certain peculiarities in the consumers' relationship to the main providers of medical care and the consumers' relationship to the medical care product that are important to an understanding of this market:

1. The physician is both the patient's purchasing consultant, who advises on what services are needed, and the seller of those services, typically on a fee-for-each-service basis. Even in the situation where the physician may not personally profit from the additional service, as in the ordering of hospital services, he is not usually inhibited from ordering them by any cost to himself.
2. Increasingly, the patient pays little or no direct cost out of his own pocket for a specific service because of the widespread use of insurance mechanisms and government payment.
3. The reimbursement of institutional providers of service by insurers and the government on a retroactively determined basis tends to remove the resistance of institutions to increasing costs.
4. The physician who makes the decisions about the amount of service to be given a patient is not trained to think in terms of aggregate cost and what is desirable when viewed statistically. His commitment is to the best interests of each individual patient in his charge, and this commitment can be at odds with attempts to reduce services that, for a large group of patients, would seem excessive.
5. In most hospitals, physicians not only are the major influence in cost decisions concerning individual patients but also have great influence on the growth and expansion of the institution. They have every reason to want to make their institution a better place in which to practice, and it does not cost the physician anything to have the institution expand.

6. The hospital product has been changing so rapidly in recent years that the introduction of some new and expensive technology seems always to prevent any previous productivity increases from being passed on to the consumer.
7. The patient is probably less able than in most other markets to judge his need for the services ordered for him, their quality, or their cost.

Notwithstanding these peculiarities of the medical market, there are four developments that promise improvements: (1) the further establishment of group practice prepayment plans and other health maintenance organizations; (2) the provision of more information to the consumer so that he can make better choices; (3) increasing consumer awareness of costs, and (4) using sophisticated third-party buyers of health services as proxies for the immediate consumer.

Health Maintenance Organizations

There is evidence that group practice prepayment plans have been successful in reducing unnecessary hospitalization and providing comprehensive care of good quality at reasonable cost. Various modifications of the traditional group practice prepayment plans, a considerable proportion of them proprietary, have been set up in the last year or two under the title of *Health Maintenance Organizations* (HMOs). The new legislation providing start-up money for HMOs and requiring an HMO option in health insurance plans paid for by employers will undoubtedly result in further growth and could within a few years introduce a competitive element of considerable significance into the provision of health care.

As compared with fee-for-service payment, the HMO method of financing shifts the economic motivation from provision of additional medical services to provision of fewer services. Since the individual has already paid his per capita fee, there is clearly no advantage to the HMO in giving him any more service than is required. Moreover, the physician himself, depending on the organization of the plan, may be at risk in ordering excessive services. From the consumer's standpoint, what has to be watched in such plans—perhaps particularly in those that are profit-oriented—is whether all necessary services are rendered. This form of organization will be competing with more traditional forms on the basis of cost, access to care, and continuity and quality of care.

The usefulness of HMOs does not depend on most people joining them. It depends just as much on the reaction of other health care providers to what is perceived as an important competitive threat. It is widely believed, for example, that the medical care foundation movement—with its important producer-sponsored cost and quality control potential—began in response to the threat of the HMO approach and the need to present fee-for-service medicine in a better light.

Improving Consumer Information

Another way of making the market approach work better is to give the consumer more information. Making public the deficiencies found in surveys of nursing homes and the information contained in the Medicare charge screens are steps in the right direction. An even more important step to place Medicare patients in a position to act on their own behalf would be to put the program on a "participating physician" basis. The participating physician would receive direct reimbursement in all cases and would be required to abide by the reasonable charge determinations of the carriers in all cases. In this way a person would know that if he went to a participating physician—and their names would be available—he would never have to pay more than the 20 percent coinsurance. Today, a physician can choose—procedure by procedure and patient by patient—to bill the patient directly and then can charge more than the carrier determines is reasonable. I would propose that if a physician chooses not to participate in Medicare, the payment be made to the patient based on a fee schedule set at the lower level of prevailing rates in the community and that the patient know what the plan would pay.

Also, since physicians often act on behalf of patients in the medical market, it would be helpful if they performed the purchasing agent function on a more informed basis. For example, it would be useful if a way were found to make physicians more conscious of drug pricing, since they are the ones who determine what prescription drugs are used.

Making Consumers More Cost Conscious

One approach to improved market functioning that has received a great deal of consideration is the attempt to make consumers more cost conscious at the time of purchase of health services by having them bear a part of the cost of each service. Many private and public plans now rely on deductibles, copayments, and co-insurance not only to reduce the costs to the plan but also as a form of utilization control. There is good evidence to show that substantial cost-sharing provisions in insurance plans—or for that matter the lack of insurance altogether—will reduce utilization of health services. The problem is that there is no evidence to indicate that such cost sharing is any more likely to reduce unneeded services than needed services. Nevertheless, in the absence of highly dependable review mechanisms, cost sharing may well be a necessary device for utilization control in connection with those services that to a considerable extent can be patient-initiated—for example, out-of-hospital prescription drugs and physician visits. At the same time there is good reason to doubt the effectiveness of such an approach in connection with hospital insurance, both because hospitalization is much less often patient-initiated and because of the ease with which the consumer can obtain supplementary insurance to cover any cost-sharing provisions in a basic plan.

Although cost sharing has limited usefulness, consumers have been made increasingly cost conscious as a result of health insurance premium increases. Today, to a very considerable extent, patients may be protected against the impact of costs at the time of purchase of service, but they are quite aware of the general problem of rising health service costs as a result of newspaper stories, insurance commissioner hearings, and specific rate increases in both private and government insurance plans. As a result, they exert pressure in favor of general cost control measures even though they are not strongly motivated to restrict their own use of services.

Purchasing by Third Parties

Third-party purchasing has improved the medical care market by doing more than the individual can to insist on quality standards and certain cost restraints. Frequently the results not only are of benefit to the direct clients of the third party but also have a pervasive effect on the whole health care system. Unions, employers, and government agencies have added some sophistication to the consumer side of the market. On the nongovernment side there are many examples of quality improvements and cost control arising from third-party activity: Employers and unions have organized health services, pressed hospitals to control cost, and insisted on broadened health insurance coverage to avoid incentives for hospitalization; years ago the United Mine Workers reduced the incidence of unnecessary surgical operations under their plan by requiring an independent consultation in cases of recommended surgery; Blue Cross in many states has used its power as a third-party payer to help prevent unneeded capital expenditures, promote reimbursement incentive plans, and foster utilization review; and commercial carriers today are devoting more attention than they once were to fighting rising costs through a policy of strict claims review.

GOVERNMENT INTERVENTION

As Third-Party Purchaser

Government as third-party purchaser has a role between that of other third-party buyers and direct government regulation. It uses its buying power to improve the health care product, as do other purchasers, but in those instances where the size of its payments makes them essential to providers—Medicare pays about a third of the costs of hospitals—its definitions and criteria have much the effect of direct, if limited, regulation.

Starting with the crippled children's program in 1936, the government has taken the view that it owed the people on whose behalf it was acting an assurance that the care being furnished met specified minimal standards of quality—in other words, it defined what it would buy—and increasingly it has taken the view that it has an obligation to try to hold down costs for the defined product to reasonable amounts.

Although product definition has many similarities to regulation, it is still quite a different matter than saying by law what can and cannot be done or what the public generally should be charged. Product definition, though less pervasive than direct regulation, may sometimes be more effective because it can avoid certain types of direct confrontations. The federal purchaser can take the view, for example, that a given level of quality may be good enough as a minimum standard for state X but not for the federal government acting on behalf of beneficiaries across the country.

The largest program in which the government acts as third-party purchaser is, of course, Medicare. Even though it became law in an atmosphere where there was great concern that the government not interfere in the way that medical care was provided, many important points of product definition and cost control were nevertheless included in the original legislation and significantly expanded in the amendments of 1972. The original legislation set up conditions of participation for skilled nursing homes that had a major impact in upgrading the level of care in the homes participating in Medicare. Accreditation by the private voluntary body, the Joint Commission on the Accreditation of Hospitals, was sufficient (except for the utilization review requirement) to qualify a hospital under Medicare under the original law, but small hospitals that had not been covered by the Joint Commission were all subject to government approval before Medicare participation was allowed; the minimum standards of state licensing were never considered sufficient for Medicare purposes. Independent laboratories were also subjected to special Medicare standards.

Perhaps the most impressive improvement in the provision of quality care for Medicare minority recipients was the insistence that all hospitals provide services on an integrated basis without regard to race. Then, too, Medicare set a standard of semiprivate room care for its beneficiaries so that segregation of the poor was greatly reduced; utilization review in institutions was required; and in other ways the health services product Medicare was willing to buy on behalf of its recipients was defined.

Cost considerations were not neglected. Claims review under Medicare very quickly became substantially more rigorous than in the usual private insurance operation, and from the beginning the design of the system encouraged less expensive forms of care in order to cut down hospital costs. For example, the extended care provision and the home health care provision were designed to substitute for expensive hospitalization. Specific measures of acceptable cost were developed, and a process for determining reasonable charges for physicians was systematically laid out. Also, of course, the willingness of the program to pay for physicians' services wherever performed—at home or at the doctor's office, as well as in hospitals—and to pay for all procedures, not just surgical procedures, greatly diminished the incentive for excessive hospitalization and surgery that is found in the usual type of partial insurance coverage.

In an atmosphere much more congenial to using government purchasing power as a lever for improving the quality of health care and controlling costs, many additional standards and controls were included in the 1972 Medicare legislation. By far the most important is the provision for professional review, which provides for the establishment of organizations of physicians throughout the country with the responsibility for determining the medical necessity of care and the adequacy and quality of care. The idea behind these Professional Standards Review Organizations (PSROs) is that it is possible to establish, within a range, appropriate hospital lengths of stay for many diagnoses and other norms for the treatment of common illnesses that define what care is inadequate and what is excessive. It is intended that, after these organizations are operating, Medicare and Medicaid will not buy services except as approved under the established guidelines.

The difficulties of full-scale implementation of the PSRO provision are staggering, but the intention is to start first with institutional care and presumably a limited number of common illnesses—the treatment boundaries of which can be agreed on—and to get experience with and evaluate various approaches to professional review based on explicit standards. No other country has tried to do anything like this and our experience with this approach is being watched with great interest around the world.

It is not at all certain that the net result of the PSRO experiment will be lower overall costs. Nor should this necessarily be the only measure of success. It could well be that unnecessary hospital care will be significantly reduced, but at the same time it is possible that much underutilization also will be corrected. It is also possible that the review system will introduce rigidities into the system that will tend to increase cost; more procedures may be performed under the banner of "quality"—because a PSRO has agreed they should be—without a clear demonstration that the additional procedures are result-oriented. And there could be a tendency to freeze practice at the level first approved by a PSRO, thus preventing some innovation and future cost saving.

These are real possibilities to be guarded against. But the idea of the medical profession taking group responsibility to determine what constitutes good care for the common diseases that require institutionalization—at least as a first step toward more general medical review—is an idea well worth trying. At present, a purchaser of care, even the government acting on behalf of millions of people, is not in a good position to judge whether a particular service is necessary or unnecessary or, if necessary, whether it could have been performed in a setting of less cost and intensity. If it works well, the PSRO approach should greatly simplify the life of health insurance administrators by helping them define what they should and should not be paying for.

Perhaps much more could be done with this leverage of government as third-party purchaser. For example, the first Health Insurance Benefits Advisory Council recommended in 1969 that Medicare should take the initiative in limiting reimbursement for specific procedures to physicians who are qualified to perform those procedures, not according to the licensing laws of the state but according to standards developed specifically for the purpose of deciding what should be paid for and what should not be paid for. If this approach were taken by such a major purchaser as Medicare, it would make a very fundamental change in the quality of health care in the United States and all at one stroke, without facing the issue state by state.

Although clearly useful in terms of upgrading the quality of care, third-party buyers, both government and nongovernment, have undoubtedly contributed greatly to increasing the cost of care. As already indicated, third-party cost reimbursement of providers calculated retroactively tends to remove the normal cost barriers to additional services, purchase of new equipment, and demands for higher wages. Moreover, the method leaves very little economic incentive for hospital management to conduct its internal affairs as economically and efficiently as possible. Leaving aside the Economic Stabilization Program, the basic formulas for Medicare and Medicaid and most Blue Cross plans are such that any savings made in the operation of hospitals result primarily in lower reimbursement. It would do a lot for the strengthening of market concepts if an effective incentive reimbursement formula could be devised to reward efficient management and—even more important from the cost standpoint—to reward the elimination of unnecessary care.

There has been considerable experience with incentive formulas in Defense Department contracting, and a number of efforts are being made in this direction in health, including some carefully designed experiments, but so far the results are not very promising. One problem, of course, is that it is very difficult to devise incentives that reach the physician, the most influential of the hospital decision makers. Perhaps we could at least set reimbursement rates prospectively, so that there would be a budget ceiling that all hospital decision makers would have to reckon with. Although not strictly an incentive plan, such a ceiling would certainly be an improvement from a cost-control standpoint over the present arrangement in which the full cost of budget increases is largely picked up by third parties.

The Conditional Grant

Another approach by government that has led to upgrading in health care is the conditional grant. For example, facility planning is now widespread because of the planning requirement in the Hill–Burton program. And hospitals built with Hill–Burton funds had to meet construction and safety standards.

In the health field, the conditional-grant method has also been used in support for health professional schools and their students; for the training and deployment of paramedicals; for the development of HMOs, neighborhood and family health centers, and community mental health centers; and for the prevention and control of specific categories of diseases.

This approach is different from regulation, but, like the definition of product by a third-party purchaser, it has similar results. By offering a grant as an inducement, it gets the health care system to perform in a certain way and at certain quality levels instead of directing it to do so, as in regulation.

Intervention by the Courts

At this conference we are not focusing on regulation of the personal health service industry by the courts. It is of some importance in this day of judicial activism, however, to remember that the courts are taking an interest in the health field in matters that used to be considered subject to purely private decision. The courts have challenged the bases on which physicians have been excluded from hospital privileges, thus moving the community hospital toward public accountability. The courts have challenged the restraints imposed upon group practice prepayment plans. The courts have more clearly defined the role of the hospital and its responsibility for the provision of medical care, thereby breaking down prohibitions against the so-called "corporate practice of medicine."

The area of court activity that perhaps has received the most attention relates to the growth in malpractice suits. This development has both its positive and its negative aspects. On the positive side, widespread threat of such suits has resulted in additional safeguards in hospital administration and in the practice of medicine generally, redounding to the advantage of patients. On the negative side, the tendency to perform extra tests and procedures as a protection against a suit is undoubtedly adding to the cost of the health care system.

Direct Federal Price Regulation

The most important direct federal regulation of personal health services is price control, and in this area the health field has been singled out for special attention. I would like to confine my comments to the very latest development—the proposed Phase IV regulations governing hospital price increases. The proposed formula for hospitals has the desirable features of tying together direct regulation and incentives while attempting to avoid control of details. In an area where retroactive cost reimbursement is the rule, the reasoning behind the regulation is that direct restraint is needed on the amount of increased cost arising not only from higher prices and wages but also from the enrichment and intensification of services. Not that some enrichment is not needed, but that in the absence of counterbalancing economic forces limiting the rate of introduction of enrichment, direct regulation to control that rate is needed.

Relating the control to hospital admissions rather than to the per diem costs or the cost of individual services puts a control that seems desirable on the total hospital budget and on the rate of the introduction of enrichment of services. I do see, however, a major problem in administration. Although the formula adjusts to the major variable of declining or increasing occupancy rates, and although there is an add-on for approved capital expansions, it is recognized that equitable treatment will require a large number of exceptions because of the special circumstances of individual hospitals. It may be very difficult to operate on a major exception basis in a way that does not greatly erode the objectives and that does respond within the time frame necessary for institutional planning.

A policy reservation that I have about the proposed regulation concerns the freedom given the states to substitute a rate-setting mechanism of their own for the federal provision. There is much to be said for this idea in terms of encouraging a variety of state experiments. The danger is that if the states get heavily into the business of rate setting, the pattern may be very hard to change. Because of this provision in the Phase IV regulation, the die may be cast for large-scale permanent state regulation of institutional charges in the health care field. This may turn out to be good or bad, but this aspect of the Phase IV regulation could settle an important national policy question without major attention being given to it.

State Regulation

Until the conditional grants of the Hill–Burton program and third-party purchasing by the federal government, the major intervention by government in the provision of health care services was through piecemeal state regulation, particularly through licensing laws. Licensing—the granting by government of the privilege to perform certain services to certain individuals and institutions and the denial to others of such a right—is based on the concept of protecting the public through a government guarantee of minimum standards. We have not, however, gone very far with this concept in practice. By tacit agreement, the U.S. approach to guaranteeing quality and competence in the provision of health services has been a two-level approach—very minimal reliance on licensing and very considerable reliance on the standards set by voluntary and professional organizations and institutions.

The lower level of this two-level approach, licensing (either of institutions or personnel), has been aimed at preventing only the most gross abuse or quackery. Physician licensing does not assure even the most minimum level of current competence. In general there are no requirements for relicensing, no requirements for continuing education, and no examination of current knowledge. A physician's license means simply that an individual once met certain educational and examination qualifications and that he has not since performed in such a conspicuously outrageous way that his license was revoked.

Complementary to the minimum approach taken by licensing has been the extensive effort at self-regulation by professional groups. In summary, in order to get some guarantee of quality, we don't today look at what a physician is licensed to do but at board certification, academy standards, etc. Most importantly (since even board certification represents a rather minimum statement of qualifications), we look to the peer judgment expressed in the hospital privileges granted by the medical staff of a good hospital. This is our primary system of quality determination, and it goes on with very little government intervention or sanction.

The situation in institutional licensing is quite similar. Licensing requirements have tended to focus on minimal fire, safety, and sanitation standards rather than on medical care. Even in the areas covered, licensing has usually been handicapped by small and inadequately trained inspection staffs. But, as in the case of personnel, institutions have been subject to standard setting by a variety of voluntary professional groups and third-party payers. Hospitals, for example, may need to be responsive to the standards of the Joint Commission on Accreditation, to standard setting for physician and nursing education programs, and to the standards of Medicare and various other third-party payers. A key issue for the future is how far the government should go in establishing standards tied to licensing laws and how much room should be left for self-regulation by professional groups that are not fully accountable to the public and to democratic processes. Another key issue is the possible modification of some of the guild-like features in licensing, which protect the monopolies of the professions. Licensing and medical practice laws can prove to be serious barriers to the most efficient use of medical manpower by prohibiting the performance of some activities by people who could learn to do them well without meeting the full educational and other requirements of the particular profession.

Recent Developments in the Area of State Regulation

There are three recent developments in the area of state regulation that will be a major focus of later discussions in this conference. They are (1) certification-of-need laws; (2) rate regulation; and (3) comprehensive regulation under a health authority.

There are now 23 states with certification-of-need laws designed to deal with the problems of duplication of services and overbuilding. Voluntary and semivoluntary planning mechanisms, started at the local and state levels and later encouraged by the federal government, have been struggling with these problems for some time. In 1966 the Partnership for Health Act established a network of comprehensive health planning agencies at state and local levels. The Act established statewide and areawide health planning agencies. The scope of activities of the two agencies was broad, including manpower as well as facility planning, but the focus has been basically on facilities. The agencies are advisory, with no enforcement powers, and a debate has been under way as to whether the agencies should continue as technical assistance staff chiefly making recommendations or whether they should also implement the recommendations.

The current low occupancy rate in a high proportion of hospitals and the recent rapid increases in per diem costs have created a demand for stronger action. This has led to pressure for statutory authority to directly regulate facility expansion through certification-of-need laws. The stated goals of the laws are clearly in the public interest. At the same time, however, there is concern about this approach based on experience with similar provisions in public utility regulation. Critics of public utility regulation can point to many instances where the consumer has lost because the control has been exercised in ways that prevented innovation and competitive choice. Will health maintenance organizations get the special consideration they will need as new institutions, or will these laws be used to protect old ways of doing things? Will the mere existence of certification-of-need laws prevent good proposals from being made?

There is concern about how effective the administration of the laws will be. Will the agencies get into the questions and issues at the takeoff or preplanning stage, or wait until plans are drawn and nearly irresistible pressures build up? When there is a need to cut back or combine or modify or add services, not merely to prevent further expansion, can the certification-of-need approach be effective?

Several states now provide for direct regulation of hospital rates. It is quite possible that several more will do so in the near future, partly, at least, because of the offer of the federal government in the proposed Phase IV regulation to let state regulation substitute for federal controls. In rate regulation it is necessary, of course, to take responsibility for controlling much more than the rate alone. As soon as one goes beyond the type of control the federal government has been exercising over rate *increases* and sets the basic rates by institution or class of institution, the rate-setting agency is soon dealing with the issues of quality of service, availability of service, subsidy of services that do not pay their own way, and control over growth and duplication of services.

Thus we are led to the third recent development—growing support for comprehensive regulation which, appearing under various names, aims at putting in one place authority related to access to care, the quality of care, the cost of care, and health manpower training with control over the numbers of general practitioners, specialists, and other health personnel. The reasoning behind this approach is that the various parts of the health care field are too interrelated to expect success if one agency focuses on the control of facility growth, another on the control of costs, perhaps another on the problem of the proper distribution of health manpower, and another on assuring broad access to medical care.

There are many detailed problems and policies of great interest in these comprehensive proposals involving, for example, the relationship of the regulatory body to the federal government as third-party purchaser. Does Medicare or an expanded national health insurance program just follow the variations of an essentially state-by-state regulatory system? Or does it continue to insist on having a say in what it will pay for and what it will not pay for? What is the relationship of the regulatory body to the voluntary standard-setting professional organizations and the hospital system of staff privileges that now act as the main guarantors of quality? Are state boundaries reasonable demarcation points for some types of regulation—the control of specialty slots in physician education, for example, under circumstances in which graduates trained in one state practice in another?

One type of comprehensive regulation, franchising by a general health authority, has considerable appeal in terms of the goal of making services generally available. We do not now have any institution or combination of institutions responsible for making sure that various levels of care are actually available throughout a geographical area. We have financing mechanisms that can be expanded to pay for the care that people are able to secure. But no one is actually charged with the responsibility for seeing that there is a skilled nursing home available in a given location, or a home health agency, or anything else. There are agencies that work on the problem, but nobody is responsible for seeing that the services are there. To me this is the great appeal of franchising. The hospital, for example, might hold a franchise only if it undertakes to make not only its services but also outpatient ambulatory and home care services available throughout the franchise territory. In this way, somebody at the operating level is held responsible for performance and outcome.

There are important theoretical and pragmatic concerns about franchising and comprehensive regulation generally, growing out of the history of public utility regulation and out of the inadequate state of our knowledge of health care and health care administration.

There is also a basis for considerable concern about putting so many eggs in the basket of state administration. With the exception of a few states, do most state governments really have the capacity to implement regulation by a unified health authority? Or, for that matter, do we know enough today at any level of government to carry out comprehensive regulation without running grave risk that we may do more harm than good? And a very key point to me: To whom are the regulators responsive? It is quite possible that in piecemeal regulation and in third-party buying there is more built-in resistance to provider pressure because of the more specific constituency than would be the case in comprehensive regulation. As third-party buyer, for example, a government insurance program considers its constituency to be the people in its program and it has a clear-cut responsibility to protect its beneficiaries by seeking quality care and by doing what it can about costs for a defined group of articulate payers. This client interest group provides a counterbalancing force to the pressures created by the interests of providers, a counterbalance that can be lacking when the constituency, as in the case of full-time regulators, is as diffuse as the general public.

Some Concluding Thoughts

People are ingenious, and this fact makes regulation very difficult. As we consider various forms of intervention in the health care system, I hope we will do so with proper respect for the great ingenuity that people show in responding to the signals of a system. Whether in employee reaction to the management of a large-scale enterprise, or in pupil reaction to the operation of an educational institution, or in private industry's reaction to regulation by government, one must be filled with admiration—no matter how grudging—for the ingenuity in getting around the "system" shown by those who are measured, directed, reported on, taught, or regulated.

But it is not only that people are ingenious at frustrating an understood purpose when it is contrary to their own goals and ambitions; equally interesting are the devastating results that sometimes arise from literal response to specified requirements. More often than not, what one measures in administration, one gets, so that one learns to be very careful about specifications and their implications. It is quite likely in the health care field that detailed specifications designed to ensure quality performance will have cost consequences that are not fully anticipated. On the other hand, one needs to be aware of the likelihood that detailed specifications designed to reduce cost in the health care field can be met with relative ease at the expense of quality, and with the quality reduced in ways that may be extremely hard to detect.

Given the observable fact of the great ingenuity of man in getting around law and regulation, supervision, and attempted education, it is a matter of some amazement how little attention tends to be paid to the intervening steps—the difficult steps grouped under the heading of administration—that must be taken between the expression of a goal and the achievement of that goal.

Finally, I would like to return to the point I mentioned at the beginning—that realistically we should not be choosing between the market, with its emphasis on incentives, and regulation, with its emphasis on directions and sanctions. I would guess that regulation that attempts to accomplish an objective by fiat, swimming upstream against a powerful current of opposing incentives, has little chance of success. But regulation that is consistent with or creates motivation that moves in the desired direction may be a different matter. Perhaps the task in the immediate future will be to strengthen incentives, competition, and choices and yet introduce direct regulation related to a relatively small number of major strategic points, seeking to avoid the rigidities that could develop in regulating the details of such a highly complicated system as health care delivery.

Can we design regulation that monitors a broad framework, while providing incentives within that framework for the great variety of actors in the system to work toward desired social objectives on their own? Can we preserve some of the contributions that come from self-regulation, and from the sophisticated buying of third parties? Can we gain from stimulating competition from new forms of organization such as HMOs? Can we develop greater and more accurate information for the prime consumer? Can we combine these approaches with improved direct regulation? These are a few of the questions we are facing.

No matter how we answer these specific questions, we can move ahead with important improvements in each of the areas that I have touched on. Whether or not comprehensive regulation is desirable at this time, there is no doubt that we can do better in promoting new forms of health care organization; we can expand the information available to consumers; we can use consumer concern to help control costs; third parties can do a better job of buying for their clients; we can, perhaps, more vigorously exploit the use of government as third-party payer; licensing standards can be upgraded and many other specific actions taken. We don't have to wait for someone else to act or for some totally integrated comprehensive approach. We can, and should, each of us act now within his own responsibility.

II

Regulation, More and Less

Experience with regulatory controls in other industries should provide some indication of what might be expected in the health care enterprise. In this section, Roger Noll examines some of the experience and finds that the results fall short of the optimistic projections made by those who would cast hospital services in the mold of a public utility. Paul M. Ellwood, Jr., sees a way to avoid imposition of permanent controls by encouraging further development of health maintenance organizations that could strongly compete in the health care market and thereby minimize the reasons for governmental regulation.

Panelists who discussed these papers were David Drake, Ph.D., associate director, American Hospital Association; Steven Sieverts, general director, Albert Einstein Medical Center, Northern Division, Philadelphia; Paul Ward, executive director, California Committee on Regional Medical Programs; and Lee White, J.D., White, Fine, and Ambrogne, attorneys, Washington, D.C.

ROGER G. NOLL, Ph.D.
Professor of Economics, California Institute of Technology

The Consequences of Public Utility Regulation of Hospitals

The health care delivery system is among the most extensively regulated sectors of the American economy. Professional licensure, hospital accreditation and certification, qualification requirements for federal subsidies, and governmental oversight of the third-party payer system constitute a complex set of institutional constraints on the structure and performance of the hospital industry.[1] Beginning about a decade ago, serious demands have been made—notably by some of the trade associations and professional societies in the industry—to complete the circle of regulation by establishing administrative agencies, at either the state or federal level, to subject the industry to "public utility" regulation. These pressures have yielded results: Most states have either established hospital regulation, or are considering legislation that would accomplish that end.

The purpose of this paper is to explore the causes and likely consequences of hospital regulation. Its point of departure is not the actual operation of the health care delivery system in the United States. Instead, the starting point is a growing body of literature in economics, law, and political science on the operation and performance of regulation generally. The first section presents some general observations on the factors that cause regulatory agencies to be established and that influence the outcomes of regulatory procedures. The second section describes some of the problems that seem to recur in regulated industries, and why these are probably inevitable consequences of imposing regulation. The third section applies these general theoretical and empirical observations to the specific case of the medical care delivery system and offers some conclusions about the relative merits of alternative methods of government intervention in the industry.

At the outset, several disclaimers must be made. This paper is not a defense of unrestrained private enterprise in medical care delivery. The nature of medical services probably requires some governmental interference in the market to counterbalance the difficulty most consumers would have in making informed, rational judgments about the effectiveness of alternative methods of treatment. The problem of an unfettered market is, furthermore, undoubtedly exacerbated by the fact that, due to insurance and federal subsidies, most medical costs are not borne directly by patients. This gives patients little incentive to consider costs in making decisions to obtain medical services—the problem of "moral hazard" common to insurance systems in which the insurable risk is to some degree determined by decisions made by the insured party.[2,3] Finally, even if these other problems could be neglected, society has every right to decide that certain goods and services—education, food, decent housing, medical services—are available to some minimum acceptable degree to all citizens, regardless of ability to pay.

The issue to be joined here is the choice among alternative arrangements for achieving society's objectives with regard to medical care. In particular, what aspects of medical care delivery are reasonably well served by a decentralized system relying on market incentives, and what other aspects are good candidates for some degree of insulation through centralized decision making from normal market mechanisms?

THEORETICAL MODELS OF REGULATION

The conventional wisdom on what regulatory authorities do and why they are established flows from the political attitudes of the turn-of-the-century progressive movement. According to the traditional view, the purpose of regulation is to protect society from abuses of market power and from other types of market failure that seem endemic to certain industries that supply key goods and services.[4] American society is seen as largely homogeneous, so that a clearly defined public interest exists and can be identified. The role of the regulator is to make certain that firms supplying services of great national importance serve this public interest: that market power or consumer ignorance is not used to enrich a relatively few businessmen while sacrificing the general welfare.

Regulatory institutions are argued to be necessary because in some industries competition cannot be relied on as a means for obtaining optimal price, output, and quality. This can occur for any of several reasons: Due to economies of scale, the most efficient size of a firm may be very large compared to the size of the industry (the "natural monopoly" case); wide, unpredictable fluctuations in supply or demand conditions within an industry may make it too risky to be attractive to many entrepreneurs unless they can earn abnormally high returns (the "ruinous competition" case); or the complexity of the product or service may be so great that consumers cannot reasonably be expected to make competent market judgments (the "consumer protection" case).

The forms of regulation that have evolved are enormously varied. *Public utility regulation* normally refers to controlling prices, profits, and the entry and exit of firms from the industry. In the traditional conceptualization, this form of regulation is paired with the "natural monopoly" case, i.e., a firm is prevented from exploiting its position in a market in which there are none or few competitors by forcing it to serve more customers at lower prices and profits than it would otherwise freely choose. But public utility regulation is by no means limited to natural monopolies: Interstate trucking, air transportation, and pipelines are federally regulated, and in most cities so are taxicabs. Yet all are, at least in the markets that generate most of the industries' sales, certainly no less competitive than many unregulated industries. In fact, this puzzling circumstance of extensive regulation of at least rivalrous if not competitive industries is an important source of dissatisfaction with traditional theory.

Another source of criticism of the traditional explanation is its failure to explain why entry control is a necessary component of regulation. If one purpose of regulation is to suppress prices so that monopoly profits cannot be made, then firms should not find entry into regulated markets attractive. In particular, if prices no more than just recover costs and if a firm enjoys economies of scale, the best outcome an entrant could achieve would be to sustain losses until the entrenched firm went bankrupt and then just to cover costs (and never recover the losses incurred while two firms were operating). Nevertheless, firms persistently have tried to enter virtually every regulated industry—not just the regulated competitive industries like trucking and taxi service, but also the so-called "natural monopolies," such as long-distance telecommunications and retail electric power distribution.

These dissatisfactions with traditional explanations of regulation have generated several new theoretical generalizations about its genesis and operation.

Capture Theories

The most radical theoretical proposition is that regulation is an institution proposed and supported by regulated industries as a mechanism for supplanting competition with a legal, enforceable cartel. This is the antithesis of the traditional view that regulation is established to protect consumers. Instead of an institution that forces monopolists or oligopolists to behave more or less as if there were competition, this theory pictures regulation as a means by which competitors can behave as if they were monopolists by making enforceable agreements to divide markets, reduce output, and raise profits.* The distinction is made apparent by comparing the explanations the two theories would have for the presence of regulation in any particular industry. For example, traditionalists would hold that the Federal Communications Commission (FCC) regulates the interstate telecommunications industry (which, without doing any great violence to reality, is essentially comprised of a single firm, the American Telephone and Telegraph Company) because interstate telecommunications service is a natural monopoly, and hence without regulation would have exorbitant prices. Those who favor the cartel explanation would contend that FCC is a device for preventing competition in telecommunications, being controlled by the Bell system for the purpose of maintaining its monopolistic position, prices, and profits.

Of course, politicians do not legalize cartels without a quid pro quo. Seeking re-election, politicians exact a "price" from the regulated industry—campaign contributions, and the establishment of an oversight agency that, while sympathetic to the regulated firms, can put some bounds on the behavior of the regulated that prevents cartel practices from being a political liability.[8] For example, a professional group will, according to the theory, gain the right to limit entry into its business, but only by accepting some responsibility for assuring minimum levels of competence among its members.

Political-Economic Theory

A similar but more elaborate model of regulation, based upon some rather recent ideas in economics and political science, sees the relation-

*In essentially contemporaneous studies, Kolko[5] and MacAvoy[6] first offered this theory as an explanation of the formation and development of the Interstate Commerce Commission. Recently Davis and North[7] have further generalized the theory to incorporate all coercive governmental institutions that create wealth for some subgroup of the population.

ship between regulators and regulated firms as more complex and dynamic. Like the traditionalists, those who subscribe to this political–economic theory assume that regulators try to serve some concept of the general public interest, rather than act as conduits for the interests of regulated firms. The problem regulators face is to identify this general public interest in a milieu in which information is uncertain, expensive, and biased, and in a society which contains numerous groups whose interests are conflicting rather than harmonious.[9]

The political–economic theory focuses on the success indicators available to regulators to assess their own performance. To a private enterprise, the best indicator of success is usually the firm's long-term profitability, or perhaps its sales. To a district attorney, it probably is convictions won; and to a politician, continued re-election.

To a regulatory authority, several success indicators are available. First is the extent to which its decisions are overridden by appeals to the courts. Second is the response of legislators to agency decisions: Do they pass bills that change an agency's decision, and do they react favorably to proposals to increase the authority and the budget of the agency? A third success indicator is the performance of the regulated industry. A cataclysmic service failure, such as the northeast power blackout of the mid-1960s, is likely to be blamed at least in part on the regulators, as is financial failure by several firms in the industry (such as has occurred in the railroad industry).

All three success indicators lead to serious biases in regulatory outcomes. Obviously, the fear of financial and service failures creates an incentive to promote the interests of the regulated firms. Healthy profits prevent financial catastrophes, and provide funds for rapid adjustments in industry operations if service should prove seriously inadequate.

More subtle is the bias inherent in the methods by which agencies collect information for reaching decisions and by which groups dissatisfied with agency decisions appeal to the courts or the legislature for a reversal. This bias arises from the costs of dealing with the regulatory system. Being represented in a regulatory proceeding is expensive. Proceedings can drag on for years when an important issue is at stake, and maintaining adequate representation can involve heavy use of expensive professionals—lawyers, engineers, economists, etc. Then, once a decision has been reached, appeals to the courts—requiring more experts—and to congressmen—certainly made more effective by campaign contributions—generate even more costs. An individual or an organized group (a firm, a trade association, a union) wishing to affect regulatory outcomes must be prepared to defray these costs of dealing with regulators, fighting court cases, and lobbying politicians. If a group is not already organized (for example, the nonexistent Association of Interstate Air Travelers), the costs of entering the regulatory process are even higher, for it must become organized in order to put together effective representation. In order for any group or individual to find entering the regulatory process worthwhile, it must expect its benefits to exceed these battle costs.

In general, the larger a group, the more expensive it is for the group to become organized to represent its members in an adversary process. And, in general, an individual is more likely to join a voluntary association if his stake in the service provided by the association is high and if the interest group of which he is a member is small enough so that his participation has an important effect on the success of the association.[10] Thus, an adversary system is more likely to be entered by a small group with a large per capita stake in the issue at hand than by a large group with a small per capita interest.

Obviously, regulated firms have a great deal at stake in regulatory proceedings, and they will choose to be effectively represented. A few customer groups who use a service extensively may also be organized and enter the process, such as a local government whose jurisdiction is about to be abandoned by a railroad or a manufacturing trade association whose members' product is about to be subjected to a freight rate increase. The stake of the general public may be even greater than any of these groups, but it is diffused over a large number of unorganized individuals. To a single consumer, any one regulatory issue is likely to be far down the list of public concerns. A consumer is unlikely to cast votes or make campaign contributions on the basis of an Interstate Commerce Commission (ICC) decision on railroad freight charges, or even to pay a few dollars to support a Washington lobbyist who will represent consumer interests before ICC. Consequently, the information presented to a regulatory authority during its deliberations is likely to come almost exclusively from special interests. In addition, only these special interests will usually pose a serious threat to appeal the agency's decision to the courts or the legislature.

All of these factors cause regulators to devote most of their attention to the effects of their policies on regulated firms and other well-represented special interest groups. First, the information flowing to the agency will be systematically biased against unrepresented groups as a natural consequence of the adversary system. Second, to minimize the chance of being overturned by the courts or the legislature, the agency will be inclined to make decisions that somewhat favor represented groups. This reduces the chance that a decision will be appealed by giving a represented group something to lose if the outcome of the appeal is unfavorable. If more than one group is well-represented on a particular issue, the agency will first engage in excruciatingly long proceedings to gather information and make a decision. This makes participating in the process even more costly, so that some groups may go bankrupt and drop out, and also postpones the day when the inevitable appeal must be fought. When the decision is finally reached, the agency will seek a compromise between the well-represented groups, giving them all some stake in the decision, which reduces the incentive anyone will have to appeal, and improves the agency's ability to defend its actions as "fair."

Legislators play an important role in the regulatory process. The legislators, being elected, are seen by regulators as an important embodiment of the public will. Yet the contact regulators have with the legislature is generally restricted to a few members of subcommittees that oversee the agency's program and budget—a relatively small proportion of the total legislature. Policies that contribute to the re-election of a few subcommittee members may not necessarily be those that could gain majority support in the legislature, but they may be instituted in any event through the informal relations between regulators and subcommittee members.* To a regulator, no practical distinction among pressures exerted by a legislator can be made on the basis of the legislator's motive, whether it be the improved efficiency of the regulated sector, the welfare of his constituents, or the profits of a contributor to his re-election campaign. In addition, the extent to which legislators can respond to special interest pleadings is greater in regulatory affairs than in the normal legislative process since the latter creates a more complete public record. For all these reasons, the subcommittee member is likely to be a very imperfect reflection of the balance among all interests in a regulatory issue, yet he is the only such indicator usually available to the agency.

EMPIRICAL OBSERVATIONS ON REGULATORY OUTCOMES

The traditional and revisionist theoretical propositions outlined above have quite different implications for the actual performance of the regulated industry. The traditional view predicts that regulation will cause prices to be lower than they would be without regulation, that to some degree regulation will eliminate some of the inefficiency due to monopolistic business practices.

The theory that regulation is a device to create a cartel has the op-

*For a description of this process vis-à-vis the National Labor Relations Board, see Scher.[11] More generally, see Wildavsky.[12]

posite prediction. A regulated industry would be characterized by higher prices, higher profits, and less output than would prevail without regulation. The political-economic theory embellishes the cartel theory, making similar predictions when only the regulated industry is represented in the regulatory process, but going on to predict that in conflict situations the regulators will go to some lengths to strike compromises among various represented groups. This is the case even though the consequences of the decision may be inefficient industry operations and higher prices to consumers.

Although the verdict is far from complete, the economics literature provides some revealing findings about the accuracy of these predictions. Economists have analyzed demand and cost conditions in several regulated industries and numerous pricing and profit decisions by regulatory agencies. Except in the case of the regulation of natural gas prices at the wellhead, no depressing effect of regulation on prices has been found. For example, retail electric and gas prices do not differ between the group of states that regulates retail power and the group that does not.[13,14] Airline fares in the intrastate markets in California, where minimum price regulation has not been practiced, are less than half the fares charged in interstate routes of similar length and passenger density that are regulated by the Civil Aeronautics Board (CAB).[15] Pipeline tariffs in regulated interstate markets are not only higher than in the unregulated intrastate markets, but apparently in some cases even somewhat higher than an unconstrained *monopolist* would charge.[16]

Natural gas field prices are the main exception, being held considerably below the best estimates of the prices that would prevail in a competitive, unregulated market. But the explanation follows from the fact that the buyers of gas at the wellhead—the pipelines—are themselves regulated. Here the relevant regulatory authority, the Federal Power Commission (FPC), is faced with the classic dilemma of arbitrating a conflict of interest between regulated groups. The response of FPC to this dilemma was, first, to refuse to regulate the industry until forced to do so by Congress and the courts, and second, to take years to make the initial decision as to how gas prices would be regulated. The resulting situation—a reduction of prices below the cost of supplying new gas—has not benefited consumers. To the contrary, prices set below the costs of new gas cause as troublesome inefficiencies as the artificially high prices charged by a monopoly. Below-cost prices have fostered uneconomically profligate use of the known reserves of the only fossil fuel that does not create serious environmental problems, have caused shortages that prevent new customers from gaining access to gas who would be willing to purchase it at a price high enough to justify opening new reserves, and have threatened existing customers with the possibility that their principal home fuel supply will disappear if the growing gas shortage causes the supplies of their retailer to be cut off.[17]

Thus the empirical evidence clearly contradicts the traditional view of regulation. Whatever regulators, do, they apparently do *not* in general reduce prices below the level that would otherwise prevail due to imperfectly competitive markets. At the same time, few studies have found any tendency of regulated firms to earn exorbitant profits. Returns to equity in regulated industries are for the most part below returns in other sectors of the economy; the common stock in regulated firms rarely has shown a long-term tendency to rise as rapidly as stock prices generally. These observations mean one of two things: Either regulation performs no function at all (that is, it has no effect on prices or profits because regulated industries are sufficiently competitive to hold these to reasonable levels) or regulation succeeds, not in lowering prices so that profits will resemble those in competition, but instead in raising costs so that the potential profitability of monopoly pricing is eroded away. A further examination of some other activities of regulators indicates that the latter is more likely to be the case.

Consumer Cross-Subsidization

One important regulatory policy that erodes the profit of monopoly pricing is the use of the price structure as an elaborate tax-subsidy scheme.[18] Regulators will permit monopoly pricing in profitable markets, but then force regulated firms to offer services in uneconomic markets that would be abandoned without regulatory intervention. Telephone service, electric power, and transportation are all priced with this consumer cross-subsidization in mind.

As mentioned before, prices are substantially lower in the California intrastate airline market than for similar interstate routes regulated by CAB. Yet interstate airlines do not earn especially high profits. One reason is that CAB has forced them to serve numerous cities that generate so little air traffic that to serve them is highly unprofitable.[19,20] Thus, the air traveler flying between two large cities—say, from Chicago to New York—not only pays for the cost of his flight, but he also pays part of the costs of flying another passenger between two smaller cities.* CAB, like other regulatory agencies, has justified consumer cross-subsi-

*Several years ago a regional air carrier ran advertisements in the *New York Times* that began with the highly relevant query: "What is Ozark doing in New York?" The answer, of course, is that CAB was trying to find a way for Ozark Air Lines to make up the losses from being in Joplin and Fort Leonard Wood.

dization on the grounds that the "national interest" requires that as many cities as possible be provided airline service, and that this is a more important objective than running an efficient national airline system. Critics of this policy respond that passengers on profitable routes, having no greater interest than does society generally in subsidizing service to small towns, should not be forced to bear the entire burden of the subsidy, assuming it is justified. They also question whether subsidies should be paid, pointing out that nowhere in CAB's legislative mandate is it directed to maximize the number of cities offered service.

The historical development of cross-subsidization by CAB illustrates the interplay between regulatory policymaking and interest groups. Initially, in response to pressure from representatives of less populous areas, Congress favored service to cities generating little traffic and provided subsidies, both indirectly through mail contracts and directly through CAB, to achieve that end. The airlines also favored the maintenance of unprofitable routes since regulation limited their profits to a fixed "fair" return on investment. The more routes flown, the greater the investment and allowed profit of an airline, and the better the prospects for future growth, investments and, hence, profits. As the nation's population became more concentrated in large urban centers, Congress looked with decreasing favor on the airline subsidy, directing CAB to work towards eliminating it. Yet many congressmen wanted service to their constituents in small cities to continue, as did the local governments and major businesses in these areas as well as the airlines. Cross-subsidization satisfied all these groups, at the expense of the passenger on major trunk routes who was unorganized and unlikely to respond to a hidden tax on air fares (from whence came the cross-subsidy) by making campaign contributions, casting ballots in congressional elections, or entering court appeals to bend policy more in his favor.

Producer Protection

The price structure can also be used by regulators to subsidize certain producers as well as particular groups of consumers. Regulatory agencies often set prices designed to prevent low-cost firms or industries from capturing business from high-cost competitors. Most often this occurs when alternative technologies have differing costs for each of several categories of service and the regulators decide not to let the firms employing these technologies specialize according to the service that each technology can offer with greatest efficiency.

Surface transportation is an interesting case in point.[21] Railroads, water carriers, and trucks usually face entirely different costs for providing a given service in a given market. If boats, trucks, and trains were to be used to best advantage, all would charge a price related to cost for each service, and shippers would then choose among transportation modes according to their relative efficiency. Yet the Interstate Commerce Commission, in an attempt to preserve for each mode some of the market for each type of shipment, often sets prices at the same level for all modes and requires that firms as "common carriers" accept shipments at those prices. Sometimes the price is below the cost of the high-cost mode so that firms are forced to accept shipments that do not cover costs, even though another firm using a different transportation technology could earn a profit on the same shipment at the same price. Sometimes the price is high enough so that all three technologies can cover costs, including the technology with the highest cost.

This practice is defended on the grounds that the national interest demands a "balanced" transportation system, giving as many shippers as possible a choice of transportation modes. The concept of unregulated monopolization of a market by a particular firm is implied to be equivalent to the concept of regulated monopolization of a market by an industry. For instance, a price decision will be said to prevent monopolization of a service by trucks. But, were it not for regulation, trucking would be a competitive industry; furthermore, trucking is regulated, which—in theory at least—is supposed to afford protection against monopolization in any event.

The argument against this policy is simply that regulation prevents shippers from capturing the benefits of a lower cost service because it breaks the connection between cost and price. Even if the national interest does require continuation of a service or preservation of a firm that customers do not want to patronize, the burden of maintaining it should not fall on shippers who favor services that are profitable, but on society generally.

Influencing Technological Change

By controlling prices, profits, and entry in an industry, regulatory agencies also control the rate and pattern of technological change. In particular, regulatory agencies have delayed or prevented many beneficial technological innovations and have promoted or permitted many others that were not justified.[22]

Thwarting a promising innovation frequently occurs when a technological change threatens to shift substantial business from one regulated firm to another or to cause the profits of a regulated industry to decline. The Federal Communications Commission provides several examples of this behavior: the long-standing prohibition (recently reversed) of foreign attachments—i.e., devices made by someone other than the American Telephone and Telegraph Company (AT&T)—to the switched telephone network; the decade-long delay in authorizing a domestic communications satellite; and the restrictions on the development of pay-television and cable television.[23] In all cases the new technology promises to offer new services that consumers have demonstrated a willingness to pay for, and old services at a substantial reduction in cost. Yet in all cases those who would own and profit from development of the new technologies differ from those who own and profit from the old: foreign attachments and domestic satellites threaten the Bell monopoly, pay-TV and cable TV threaten the highly profitable tight oligopoly enjoyed by VHF (very high frequency) television stations (channels 2 to 13) in large cities, as well as what remains of the motion picture and live theatre industries. Even though neither AT&T nor VHF broadcasters would be forced out of business by a more permissive policy, the fact that they would be damaged due to the loss of some of their insulation from competition is regarded as sufficient cause by FCC to prevent, delay, or severely limit an economically warranted technological advance. Meanwhile the resources of the potential entrants for dealing with regulators, the Congress, and the courts are far fewer than those of the entrenched firms—partly because they have no profitable existing markets to finance their operations and partly because many of those who would profit from new technology have yet to emerge.

Transportation regulation also abounds with similar examples. For instance, the piggybacking case illustrates a penchant for tinkering with technology by ICC. The ICC Rail Form A specifies the minimum revenue that a railroad flatcar must earn when fully loaded. When the railroads introduced piggybacking, or carrying truck freight on a railroad flatcar, ICC insisted that the piggyback flatcars satisfy the Rail Form A revenue requirements. This decision forced the railroads not only to charge a higher price for piggybacking than they would otherwise have levied, but also to adopt an inferior method of providing the service. In providing piggyback service, the railroads faced a two-dimensional technical decision. The first concerned the length of the flatcar: Should it be large enough to carry one or two truckloads? The second concerned the part of the truck to be carried: Should the entire truck-trailer be carried (including the wheels) or just the freight container? The lowest cost alternative for most railroads was to carry only the container and to use short flatcars that could carry only one truckload. Securing a container to a flatcar is easier than securing a wheeled trailer, and the shorter car is more stable on steeply banked roadbeds, can manage the sharpest curves in tunnels without scraping the walls, is compatible with normal railyard switching equipment, and requires no excess capacity if an odd number of trucks is to be carried. But by insisting that Form A rates be used, ICC prevented the low-cost method from being adopted, since the Form A revenue requirement for a one-truck car was far too high to induce truckers to use piggybacking. Because the price per truck on a double-truck car could, according to Form A, be half the rate on a single-truck car, the railroads were forced to adopt the former despite the fact that to do so necessitated redigging tunnels, rebanking curves, and redesigning switchyards. And since the price on a flatcar transporting whole trailers could not differ from the price on flatcars transporting only the freight container, railroads were legally barred from giving the trucking industry a financial incentive to use trucks with removable containers, even though the cost savings from flatcars for removable containers were more than enough to make up for the extra costs of making trailer containers removable. Thus, the full cost advantage of the piggyback innovation could not be captured, and that which was captured could not be fully reflected in prices. This served partly, but not wholly, to inhibit the innovation. Rails did capture some long-distance traffic from trucks and waterways, but less than was economically warranted by the economics of the innovation. And in the process, the distribution of business and profits among transport modes was upset less than would otherwise have been the case. The main loser was the consumer, since commodity prices subsequently included unnecessarily high freight costs.

Another source of the reluctance of regulators to permit innovation arises from the uncertainty inherent in change. A new technology may be *expected* to produce great benefits, but usually there is a *chance* that it can cause a deterioration in some aspect of service. The agency faces an asymmetric penalty to making mistakes in such circumstances. Preventing a technology that would have been worthwhile may generate criticism, but at least the criticisms will be based on conjectural information on the uncertain potential of the new technology. And at least some of those who would have benefited from the technology will not be a source of criticism since they will not have realized their potential gains. On the other hand, adopting a technology that is not successful leads to the more informed, diverse criticism of hindsight. The agency will share the blame for service failure, and will be criticized by those who lost business because the new technology was adopted.

Furthermore, associated with even an unsuccessful technology that is adopted will be some firms and workers whose welfare depends on its continued use. These groups represent one more voice to be reckoned with by the agency.

These asymmetric costs of mistakes give agencies an incentive to exercise excessive caution when dealing with technological innovations. They will tend to block or to retard innovations that threaten entrenched interests. Even when the new technology is proposed by entrenched interests and is not expected to redistribute income against any of the agency's well-represented clients, they will tend to delay decisions in an attempt to acquire more information and thereby reduce uncertainties about the possible detrimental consequences of an innovation.

Regulation-Induced Inefficiency

The presence of regulation, by altering the incentives faced by firms, also damages the efficiency of their operations. First, the profit ceiling imposed upon regulated firms is usually based upon costs. In trucking, for example, firms may earn profits up to a fixed proportion of total costs, while in telecommunications firms may earn profits equal to a fixed percentage of the depreciated book value of their capital investments. Of course, this means that a firm can earn greater profits only if it incurs greater costs, which blunts the normal business incentive to produce output at the minimum possible expense.[24]

Second, the policies of regulators that force firms to operate in uneconomic markets, that protect inefficient firms from competition, and that retard technological developments that threaten to redistribute business among firms create an atmosphere among entrepreneurs that is not conducive to innovation, creativity, and efficiency. Since the second world war, the railroad industry has been roundly criticized for poor management, and certainly judging from developments in rail transport in Europe and Japan, the criticisms appear to have some foundation.

The decline in railroad management followed shortly after ICC was given the responsibility to regulate trucking. In the absence of regulation, the expected consequence of the technological development of trucking in the 1920s and 1930s would have been some specialization of services by each mode and some retaliatory innovation by the rails. But ICC policies of preventing truck–rail competition and of forcing the rails to continue shipping some commodities and serving some communities after the rise of trucking had made these inefficient for rail service must have played some role in undermining the entrepreneurial spirit in the railroad business.

Finally, attempts to regulate competition inevitably lead to a "tar-baby" effect of increasingly complex regulatory constraints.[25] When regulators protect a weak competitor or generate extra profits for cross-subsidization in a competitive market, they generally succeed more in changing in the arena of competition rather than in preventing it. Disallowed from competing through price reductions, firms will turn to improvements in service quality—improvements that, without price controls, consumers would not be willing to pay for—as a mechanism for obtaining more customers. In the airline industry, for example, high prices on profitable routes have lead to more frequent flights (with fewer passengers per flight) and increases in in-flight services.[26] Since these service improvements increase costs, they erode the profits for cross-subsidization. To preserve unprofitable routes, CAB must impose restrictions on service competition—by arbitrating mutual reductions in flights among competing airlines, by insisting that airlines charge for movies and alcoholic beverages that initially are given away, and even by defining the maximum square inches of a tourist-class seat. And, as each new avenue of competition is closed off, creative businessmen discover another, the "piano bar" being the latest. This unending sequence of innovative competition and regulatory response is the counterpart in regulation of Brer Rabbit's uncommunicative, sticky stranger.

The Costs of Regulation

The preceding discussion reveals what regulation does and does not do: Generally, regulators do not prevent monopoly prices. In fact to some extent they encourage monopoly prices as a kind of sales tax to finance "good works" by regulated firms in the form of subsidies to uneconomic services, firms, and technologies. (We can all give thanks that ICC was not established in the 1860s, or else we probably would still receive some of our mail by Pony Express.)

The discussion as yet contains no indication of the magnitude of the inefficiencies attendant to regulation. Some work has been done in this area, although the results are by no means complete.

First, the costs of operating the major federal public utility regulatory agencies—the Securities and Exchange Commission (SEC), FCC, ICC, CAB, and FPC—probably approach $1 billion annually. The agencies have budgets of about $25 million each, and the firms that are regulated probably spend several times as much in dealing with the agencies, the courts, and Congress on regulatory matters. Much of this expenditure is for pro forma, unproductive activities.[27]

Second, several estimates indicate that the costs of regulation in terms of the losses in efficiency of regulated firms is even higher than the direct cost of running the institution. For example, ICC regulation of surface freight transportation has been estimated to cost $5 billion annually, due to the shift from lower cost to higher cost modes caused by inconsistent cost–price relationships among the modes.[26] The costs of an irrational pricing structure in air transportation probably are of a similar magnitude.[20] Thus, the unnecessary costs created by regulators are not minor; indeed they may account for 25–50 percent of the revenues of regulated firms.[28] It is at least open to debate whether or not the American public, if given the opportunity, would cast a favorable vote on the proposition that the stability and uneconomic services resulting from regulation are worth this cost.

The inefficiencies attendant to regulation provide an explanation for why regulators are compelled to control entry—an explanation that, as remarked before, eludes traditional theory. If prices in some regulated markets produce profits above those that are necessary to keep a firm in business in the long run so that cross-subsidies can be paid, inefficient firms can be preserved, regulation-induced costs can be covered, or inferior technologies continued in use; then regulators must control entry. High profits, or the potential for profit with more efficient operation, will attract new firms. Their uncontrolled entry would lead to a loss of business by the firms internally subsidizing losing markets, or for some other reason favored by the regulators. To protect inefficient operations and cross-subsidies, further division of the market through entry must be prevented.

IMPLICATIONS FOR HOSPITAL REGULATION

Quite obviously, the preceding arguments hardly lead to happy conclusions about the consequences of public utility regulation of hospitals. The two principal conclusions to be extracted from the above discussion are (1) regulation tends to protect regulated firms whenever competition or technological change threatens established positions within the industry, and (2) regulators see the purpose of the price structure as providing a mechanism for taxing some groups and subsidizing others, rather than as a mechanism for offering incentives to buyers and sellers to rationalize choices among inputs, outputs, and technologies. Thus, if the pattern extends to public utility regulation of hospitals, the following results could be expected to obtain: (1) resistance by regulators to innovations in medical care delivery systems (such as prepaid group health plans) regardless of their merits; (2) substantial consumer cross-subsidization and producer protectionism in the price structure; and (3) persistent upward drift in prices toward monopolistic levels in order to finance subsidies and inefficiencies created by regulation.

The preceding description is reminiscent of the current situation in the hospital industry. The medical economics literature is replete with claims that existing regulatory practices in the industry produce all of these results. Professional licensure and hospital certification institutionalize existing medical technology, in part because they prevent using different combinations of inputs to provide a given service and in part because medical malpractice judgments are to some extent based upon the standards for licensure and certification.[29,30] Similarly, the straightforward cost-reimbursement system by which third-party payers, particularly Blue Cross and the federal government, determine how much hospitals should be paid eliminates financial incentives to be efficient or to introduce cost-saving innovations.[1]

Those who favor even greater regulation of hospitals argue as follows.[31] First, the failures of regulation in other areas are irrelevant to the hospital case because hospitals are almost exclusively nonprofit institutions. Second, regulation is necessary because the unusual relationships among hospitals, doctors, patients, and payers prevents normal market incentives from working. Third, the problems of oversensitivity to regulated firms discussed above are said to be mitigated by the presence of strong, well-organized groups on the other side of the market. Fourth, the failures of the incomplete, weak regulation that hospitals now experience are due to the fact that regulation of hospitals has not been complete enough and has not been enforced by strong administrative agencies.

Nonprofit Status

The nonprofit status of hospitals is, in reality, not of major consequence.

First, the nonprofit status of hospitals is not unique. Nonprofit, governmentally owned enterprises are common in the electric utility and local transportation industries. Although nonprofit firms tend to charge somewhat lower prices, this is largely explained by their favored tax status. The main beneficiaries of nonprofit status appear to be employees, since nonprofit firms apparently pay higher wages.[32,33] Nonprofit firms are also somewhat less prone to practice price discrimination.[33,34] Nevertheless, these differences among profit and nonprofit enterprise in other regulated industries are small.

Second, most of the inefficiencies due to regulation arise from the policies of the regulators, not of the regulated firm. Cross-subsidization, producer protection, and overly cautious attitudes about innovation all are aided and abetted, if not initially conceived, by the regulators.

Third, the profit–nonprofit distinction probably has far less impact on most operating decisions than operators of nonprofit institutions suppose. The profit-orientation assumed to characterize private enterprise is a shorthand generalization of something far more complicated. A firm, like any other organization, only has goals to the extent that the people who control it have goals. The profit orientation of a firm reflects the profit orientation of equity holders, which is to say that those in control of an institution adopt policies in their own interest. A nonprofit institution is also run by individuals interested in their own welfare.

Since the types of people who control nonprofit institutions may differ from those who run profit-making enterprises, nonprofit institutions do behave differently in some circumstances than profit-oriented ones.[35] But this behavior is not crucial as far as predicting the consequences of regulation is concerned. Some studies have examined the proposition that hospitals are organized to some degree to benefit doctors.[36,37] If hospitals are a "doctors' cooperative," their nonprofit orientation is a legal reality but practical fiction, and hospital regulation will be essentially regulation of a profit-oriented group of doctors.

Other studies have postulated different motives for those who operate nonprofit institutions. For the most part, these differences are over how the returns from profitable activities are to be spent. A profit-seeking organization will use these returns to pay equity holders or to reinvest in other profitable activities. A nonprofit organization will usually spend these returns on unprofitable activities: on unnecessary expenditures (such as on capital investments that are monuments to the officers), on providing unremunerative services (the counterpart to cross-subsidization in a regulated firm), on improving product quality beyond the level that its customers are willing to pay for, or simply on rising costs resulting from paying too little managerial attention to cost-efficiency.[38,39,40] What is unlikely to differ significantly between profit and nonprofit enterprises is the price of a profitable service. In fact, the nonprofit enterprise, to the extent it operates in an unregulated and uncompetitive market, has a tendency to engage in the same inefficient practices that regulation creates for the profit-making institution.

The desire for stronger regulation on the part of hospitals is certainly consonant with the manner in which nonprofit institutions tend to exhaust their profits. Both nonprofit and for-profit institutions seek to protect themselves from competition, but for different reasons. To the for-profit institution, insulation from competition increases the profitability and reduces the financial risk of investment in the industry. To the nonprofit institution, the additional revenue-earning potential of insulation from competition expands the financial resources for doing "good works." To the indigent, the victim of an exotic illness that is expensive to treat, and the trustee wishing to construct the modern version of a pyramid in his own name, the uses of profits by the regulated nonprofit hospital have enormous value, and certainly a legitimate case can be made that nonprofits make better use of monopoly prices than do profit-making institutions. But for the broad range of hospital services, both types of institutions yield similar results: monopoly prices in excess of costs to the extent that market conditions permit. And with regulation, the outcomes become even more similar as the profit-making institution is induced by the regulators to engage in the same type of internal tax-subsidy policies and inefficiencies that tend to characterize the operations of the nonprofit institution.

Consumer Powerlessness

Regulation is also said to be needed because it is necessary to deal with the unusual phenomenon in medical care in which the patient receives the service, the doctor chooses the hospital, and the insurer pays the bill. The basis of the argument is the observation that nowhere in the system is an individual decision made with costs in mind.[2,41] Consequently, runs the argument, regulation is necessary to overcome the absence of an incentive for cost reduction.

The problem with this argument is that the conclusion is a *non sequitur*. Nowhere in our experience with regulation is there the slightest indication that regulation can instill more attention to costs than regulated industries would have on their own.

The interest in applying increasingly tighter controls on entry into the hospital industry provides an interesting point of departure to illustrate the problems with using regulation as a mechanism to control costs. Obviously, rapidly expanding capacity and dwindling occupancy rates are not, by themselves, the objectives of hospital administrators. They reflect individual decisions not to maximize beds, but to provide medical services at financially remunerative prices. The persistent overinvestment in facilities is based upon the belief that in the long run hospitals will not fail financially. This belief is surely going to be reinforced the greater the extent to which third-party payers dominate the market and government intervenors determine prices through strict cost-reimbursement formulas.

Suppose in this milieu a strict prohibition on further expansion of capacity is enforced. This in no way changes the motives and the financial environment in which former decisions to expand capacity had been made. It simply means the beds can no longer be a major resultant of the interaction between these motives and financial conditions. The inadequate incentives for cost-reduction and rational pricing would remain, as would the potential to use the price system to collect capital for other unnecessary expenditures besides unused beds. Controlling the number of beds will simply turn the attention of hospital administrators to other, perhaps even less desirable expenditures. Thus is the regulatory tar-baby conceived. Regulators will find their attempts to force efficiency upon a recalcitrant industry as leading only to ever more detailed and expensive regulation, prohibiting a lengthening string of unnecessary expenditures, but with no apparent long-run success in dealing with the general problem of rising costs.

Fair Representation

Another proregulation argument is that those who purchase hospital services are well-enough organized to provide a countervailing force to hospitals before an administrative agency. Certainly this argument is not without substance. Organizations such as Blue Cross, private insurers, the Social Security Administration, and other major payers are organized to plead their cases before a regulator. Their presence, according to the theoretical arguments advanced above, should make regulatory outcomes more of a compromise than if regulators only talked to representatives of hospitals. Unfortunately, this does *not* mean that regulation will produce a better outcome than even the present system.

The position of those not represented by a third-party payer will probably be weakened under regulation. Today such patients face a multiplicity of hospitals with some degree of independence in making decisions on prices and service quality. Although hospital "shopping" is admittedly difficult, it nevertheless is possible for some consumers. With regulation, decisions on prices will be centralized, to be decided in an adversary process in which these patients are unlikely to be represented. Whatever the value of the minimal shopping and bargaining among hospitals that now takes place, it will be lost under regulation.

Probably more important is the change that regulation will make in the bargaining relation between major third-party payers and hospitals. Here the importance of independent decision making among hospitals is significant, for third-party payers *can* deal with hospitals individually and provide some incentives for cost reduction if they so choose. Regulation allows hospitals to bargain as one before the regulatory authority, thereby avoiding the possibility that a more efficient hospital will strike a special bargain that undercuts the position of other hospitals. In fact, one reason advanced by hospitals for the necessity of regulation is the ability of Blue Cross and the Social Security Administration to obtain "preferential" prices.[42] The hospitals expect that a regulatory system that allows them to bargain as a unit will produce a better result for hospitals than does a decentralized system. Further, they see a possibility for what appears to them to be a desirable cross-subsidy: charging equal prices to insured and uninsured patients even though the latter are more likely to default on payments and, therefore, are more costly to serve.

Finally, the interests of insured patients and insurers do not necessarily coincide, which makes third-party payers imperfect representatives of the interests of even insured consumers. Health insurance does not pay the same proportion of all hospital costs, so that insurers will benefit from cross-subsidization of highly insured treatments by less-insured ones. Furthermore, as long as profit-oriented insurance companies can forecast accurately, they are not necessarily affected adversely by price increases. The demand for hospital insurance depends upon the financial risk of facing hospitalization without coverage. Rising hospital prices cause insurance rates to rise, but they also increase the risk of self-insurance. Depending upon the consumer's degree of risk aversion, and the sensitivity of his demand for hospital services to prices, rising hospital fees could lead to an increased demand for insurance, thereby benefiting insurers. And in states that regulate insurance by requiring that underwriting profits have some fixed relation to premiums and reimbursements, rising hospital costs can be the only mechanism, short of epidemic, for increasing insurance company profits.

Regulatory Failure

That regulation of the quality of health care has failed to stem inflation in hospital costs* and to maintain satisfactory standards of care

*For a while, the price control programs initiated in 1971 moderated inflation in the entire economy, including hospital care. This experience has virtually no relevance to public utility regulation: Price controls are temporary, are applied across the board to all industries (insulating the administrators from much of the special-interest pressures affecting regulators), and are administered by an agency having no responsibility to maintain stability in any particular industry.

is generally agreed. That this justifies further regulation is dubious.

The preceding arguments suggest that a central cause of the problems besetting the hospital industry is the set of institutional arrangements insulating hospitals from market incentives. Imposing public utility regulation upon the existing system is probably the only step that could be taken to make the industry even more insulated from incentives to be efficient. Any system that separates the payer from the recipient of service will be prone to inefficiencies; imposing regulation on such a system simply adds one more group whose tastes for uneconomic services and inefficient operations must be served.

Abandoning regulation is not necessarily equivalent to abandoning medical care to the quacks. If the problem with a medical care delivery system based upon cost incentives (e.g., extensive coinsurance or prepaid group health) is a tendency to utilize consumer ignorance to provide ineffective, low-quality service, a more sensible approach is to control performance directly. Various licensure, certification, and accreditation regulations in theory are designed to achieve this, but they exact too high a price in preventing innovation and in entrenching the power of specific professional groups. More effective is the regulation of health outcomes in a more consistent, comprehensive, and scientific manner than the medical malpractice suit.[43]

Generally speaking, regulation to impose minimum performance standards is more successful than public utility regulation: Airlines are safe and growing safer, despite the inefficiencies in their pricing and operations; emissions from automobiles and smokestacks are falling rapidly. This is not to say that minimum standard regulation is always sensible, efficient, and effective, but merely that some evidence can be found that it can produce noticeable results consistent with its aims.

Experience indicates that society does relatively better by centralizing quality decisions while relying upon individual, decentralized decisions, based upon market incentives, for achieving cost efficiency. Imposing public utility regulation on the present system moves in precisely the wrong direction: It relies upon individual decision makers or homogeneous, self-interested professional groups to make decisions on the quality of service in an arena in which the consumer has no reasonable expectation of being able to judge quality, but it relies on cumbersome, centralized decision making to promote efficiency. A necessary component of promoting efficiency is introducing the threat that a bad decision will lead to financial difficulties; and a necessary component of assuring that minimum quality standards are met is to make sure that someone representing the consumer's interest has a role in passing judgment on the seller's decisions about quality. It is difficult to conceive of an institutional framework more removed from this latter model than one in which the present system is amended by grafting on public utility regulation.

ACKNOWLEDGMENTS

I am indebted to Ralph Berry, Clark Havighurst, Michael Levine, and Jeffrey Weiss for helpful comments on an earlier draft. Part of the costs of preparing this manuscript was financed by the National Science Foundation, Grant No. DA-39495.

REFERENCES AND NOTES

1. Somers AR: Hospital Regulation: The Dilemma of Public Policy. Princeton, Princeton University Press, 1969.
2. Arrow KJ: Uncertainty and the welfare economics of medical care. Am Econ Rev 53:941–973, 1965.
3. Pauly MV: The economics of moral hazard: Comment. Am Econ Rev 58: 531–537, 1968.
4. Wilcox C: Public Policies Toward Business. Homewood, Ill., Irwin, 1960.
5. Kolko G: Railroads and Regulation. Princeton, Princeton University Press, 1965.
6. MacAvoy PW: The Economic Effects of Regulation: The Trunkline Railroad Cartels and the ICC before 1900. Cambridge, Massachusetts Institute of Technology Press, 1965.
7. Davis LE, North DC: Institutional Change and American Economic Growth. Cambridge, Cambridge University, 1971.
8. Stigler GJ: The theory of economic regulation. Bell J 2 (1971).
9. Noll RG: Reforming Regulation: An Evaluation of the Ash Council Proposals. Washington, D.C., Brookings Institution, 1971.
10. Olson M: The Logic of Collective Action. Cambridge, Harvard, 1965.
11. Scher S: Congressional committee members as independent agency overseers: A case study. Am Polit Sci Rev 54:911–920, 1960.
12. Wildavsky A: The Politics of the Budgetary Process. Boston, Little, Brown & Co., 1964.
13. MacAvoy PW: The effectiveness of the Federal Power Commission. Bell J 1 (1970).
14. Moore TG: The effectiveness of regulation of electric utility rates. South Econ J (April 1970).
15. Levine ME: Is regulation necessary? California air transportation and national regulatory policy. Yale Law J 74 (1965).
16. MacAvoy PW, and Noll RG: Relative prices on regulated transactions of the natural gas pipelines. Bell J 4 (1973).
17. MacAvoy PW: The regulation-induced shortage of natural gas. J Law Econ (October 1970).
18. Posner RA: Taxation by regulation. Bell J 2 (1971).
19. Eads GC: The Local Service Experiment. Washington, D.C., Brookings Institution, 1972.

20. Keeler TE: Airline regulation and market performance. Bell J 3:394–424, 1972.
21. Friedlaender AF: The Dilemma of Freight Transport Regulation. Washington, D.C., Brookings Institution, 1969.
22. Capron WM (ed): Technological Change in Regulated Industries. Washington, D.C., Brookings Institution, 1971.
23. Noll RG, Peck MJ, McGowan JJ: Economic Aspects of Television Regulation. Washington, D.C., Brookings Institution, 1973.
24. Averch H, Johnson LL: Behavior of the firm under regulatory constraint. Am Econ Rev 52 (1962).
25. McKie JW: Regulation and the free market: The problem of boundaries. Bell J 1 (1970).
26. Phillips A (ed): Competition and Regulation. Washington, D.C., Brookings Institution (forthcoming).
27. MacAvoy PW: The formal work-product of the federal power commissioners. Bell J 2 (1971).
28. Green MJ (ed): The Monopoly Makers. New York, Grossman Publishers, 1973.
29. Carlson RJ: Health manpower licensing and emerging institutional responsibility for the quality of care. Law Contemp Probl 35:849–879, 1970.
30. Elwood PM, Jr, O'Donoghue P, et al.: Assuring the Quality of Health Care. Minneapolis, InterStudy, 1973.
31. Priest AJG: Possible adaptation of public utility concepts in the health care field. Law Contemp Probl 35:839–848, 1970.
32. Hamermesh DS: The effect of government ownership on union wages, Working Pap No. 428. Princeton, Industrial Relations Section, Princeton University.
33. Pashigian BP: Public vs. private ownership: Consequences and determinants of public ownership of local transit systems. Chicago, University of Chicago Graduate School of Business, October 1973 (mimeograph).
34. Peltzman S: Pricing in public and private enterprises: Electric utilities in the United States. J Law Econ 14:109–148, 1971.
35. Davis K: Economic theories of behavior in nonprofit, private hospitals. Econ Bus Bull 24(2):1–13, 1972 (Brookings Repr No. 239).
36. Pauly M, Redisch M: The not-for-profit hospital as a physicians' cooperative. Am Econ Rev 63:87–99, 1973.
37. Perrow C: Goals and power structures: A historical case study. In E Friedson (ed), The Hospital in Modern Societies. New York, NY Free Press, 1963, pp 112–146.
38. Lee ML: A conspicuous production theory of hospital behavior. South Econ J 38:48–59, 1971.
39. Feldstein MS: Hospital cost inflation: A study of nonprofit price dynamics. Am Econ Rev 61:853–872, 1971.
40. Newhouse JP: Toward a theory of nonprofit institutions: An economic model of a hospital. Am Econ Rev 60:64–74, 1970.
41. Reder MW: Some problems in the economics of hospitals. Am Econ Rev 55: 472–481, 1965.
42. Cohen HA: The application of the public utility model to hospitals and related institutions. Health Services Cost Review Commission, State of Maryland (mimeograph).
43. Havighurst CC: Health maintenance organizations and the market for health services. Law Contemp Probl 35:716–795, 1970.

PAUL M. ELLWOOD, JR., M.D.
Director, Health Services Research Center, InterStudy, Minneapolis

Alternatives to Regulation: Improving the Market

Early in 1970, the federal government took a few tentative but historic steps aimed at restructuring the American health industry and making it reasonably self-regulating, competitive, and more responsive to market forces. These actions were part of a larger set of initiatives that came to be known as the health maintenance organization strategy. Since then the HMO strategy has undergone a preliminary period of testing. This paper examines this initial experience in terms of the assumptions on which the strategy was based, and—in the light of that experience and the current state of health policy and politics—proposes additional steps that might be taken now to strengthen the medical market.

The ideas embodied in the HMO strategy were not new, but their endorsement and active promotion by an administration intent on restructuring the health system constituted a dramatic departure in U.S. health policy. In effect, the new policy signaled that the federal government would no longer maintain its traditional hands-off attitude toward the health industry's internal working arrangements and the incentives that govern providers, and that it intended instead to assume the role of active agent for change.

The past is replete with enlightened delivery system reforms that have come to naught, ranging from the proposals of the Wilbur Commission in the 1930s to the efforts surrounding the passage of Medicare [e.g., the Regional Medical Program (RMP) and Comprehensive Health Planning (CHP)] in the 1960s. Thus, it was optimistic, if not naïve, to presume that the modest actions of the HMO strategy could succeed in restructuring the American health system to a greater degree than has yet been achieved by any other nation in the world. Yet the gravity of the industry's problems clearly demanded that some kind of remedial action be tried. There were mounting pressures both for tighter regulatory control and for a deliberate effort to improve the health market; it seemed reasonable to assume that the providers of care would prefer the voluntary course of action set forth in the HMO strategy.

ASSUMPTIONS UNDERLYING THE MARKET APPROACH

Rather than reiterating the problems that gave rise to the HMO strategy and the specific measures proposed for its implementation, let me briefly discuss the underlying assumptions from which this market-oriented strategy emerged.[1]

In 1970, the health care delivery situation was not too different from today's circumstances. Evidence from a variety of sources, including a hard-hitting report issued by the Senate Finance Committee, pointed conclusively to the unchecked inflation in private and public expenditures for health care, and created strong political pressures for decisive action.[2] The Social Security Administration, in concert with the staff of the House Ways and Means and Senate Finance committees, had begun work on a series of amendments to Medicare and Medicaid, aimed at controlling costs largely through regulation. At about the same time, a federal task force was assembled under the leadership of Walter McNerney, president of the Blue Cross Association, to suggest ways for improving the performance of government health insurance programs.[3]

The executive branch also recognized the need for action, but was wary of imposing additional controls on a health system that, in its view, was already subject to extensive and not-too-successful regulation by both state and federal governments. Almost in desperation, leaders of the administration turned to the HMO strategy, which seemed to offer a natural solution to the problems at hand, while avoiding the unwelcome alternative of tighter and more pervasive government control.

The approach was based on the conviction that structural reform is an essential prerequisite to any long-term solution, and that mandatory change is neither desirable nor politically feasible. Even if it were possible politically to install a planned health system, it was felt that not enough is known about health needs and optimal delivery arrangements to design the ideal system. Hence, attention focused on how a process of voluntary change might be set in motion, and what incentives might be used to create a more effective delivery system.

It should be recognized that the political actions taken by the administration, Congress, and the states, in response to the inflationary ferment of the past few years, have been distinctly ambivalent in that they have embodied a mixture of incentive and regulatory strategies. This ambivalence persists and the search for tentative measures on the regulatory front to match the equally tentative efforts to restructure the health market goes on. The ideas put forth in this paper are aimed at resolving this potentially harmful conflict in the approach to be followed as we seek to improve the health industry's present unfavorable performance.

The health maintenance organization strategy grew out of certain specific assumptions that were founded on a mixture of well-established facts and observations about the existing health system, basic economic principles, and pragmatic political judgments. Those assumptions were as follows:

1. *The health industry can be restructured.* Providers will respond to appropriate federal initiatives by forming HMOs, provided that the definition of such organizations is sufficiently flexible to permit them to work out whatever internal organizational arrangements they prefer.
2. *Prepaid health care organizations providing comprehensive services to enrolled consumers will be equally effective on a national scale.* New HMOs—like existing prototypes—will reduce hospitalization and allocate such resources as primary physicians and hospital beds more efficiently than the existing health system.
3. *The competitive health market will work.* As HMOs become more numerous, competition will increase and have a positive impact on the performance of both fee-for-service providers and HMOs themselves.
4. *If HMOs succeed, the need and desire for expanded regulation of the health industry will diminish.* If new HMOs form in sufficient numbers and perform like existing prototypes, and if the competition they engender has a favorable effect on the performance of all providers, then the need for greater government planning and regulatory intervention will be minimal and political pressure for more controls will cease.

The first assumption, that providers would respond positively to appropriate incentives by forming HMOs, involved the resolution of two important issues. Should HMOs be defined precisely, or in terms of broad fundamental principles and incentives? And, what federal initiatives could elicit the desired voluntary response from providers?

It was recognized that a flexible definition could have the unfortunate effect of alienating some who otherwise might be inclined to support the HMO strategy. For instance, some advocates of prepaid group practice are convinced that such organizations can only succeed if they are modeled in terms of a specific code based on extensive operating experience, and they might oppose a definition that did not include organizational specifications.[4] Others strongly believe that consumer control is a necessary condition of health system reform, and might oppose a definition in which this was not a mandatory requirement. Still others might oppose a flexible definition because it would permit for-profit firms to establish HMOs, or because it might encourage monopolies, or because it would not guarantee physician control, and so on.[5]

However, the potential benefits of a flexible definition seemed to outweigh these risks. For one thing, by insisting that all HMOs be cast from the same classic organizational mold, it seemed likely that the opposition of organized professional groups could be neutralized, and thus that the base of HMO support among physicians and other provider groups could be broadened. Moreover, the danger of locking in the health system to a rigid organizational formula seemed implicit in a narrow definition, while a flexible one would permit and encourage organizational diversity and continuing innovation. For these reasons, it was decided that HMOs should be defined in terms of broad operating principles, and that the definition should be deliberately vague with respect to their internal structure.[6] As expected, this has been a controversial aspect of the HMO approach, and one that has never been entirely accepted by many advocates of prepaid health care. One consequence has been that state and federal enabling acts defined HMOs more narrowly and in greater detail than was originally proposed.

To encourage the formation of HMOs, a series of federal initiatives was outlined, beginning with the use of the government's persuasive influence to legitimize and promote the idea of delivery system reorganization. In the past, attempts to alter the way health care is delivered often have been effectively stifled by organized medicine's adamant opposition to structural change. Despite this traditional bias, certain trends toward greater organization in health delivery were apparent,[7] and it was felt that these trends could be accelerated by publicly endorsing new forms of delivery and by persuading providers to cooperate voluntarily in bringing about delivery system reform. There were also indications that the attitudes of rank and file physicians were softening with respect to prepaid group practice,[8] and it seemed likely that the perceived threat of increased public control over professional activities would reinforce this shift. Furthermore, the continued success of prototype HMOs in delivering care efficiently while holding down inflation, provided government spokesmen with concrete examples of what reorganization could accomplish.

In addition to legitimizing change, it was decided that specific legislative measures should be promoted to encourage and implement delivery system reform. These included the elimination of state legal barriers to HMO formation;[9] making available various forms of government grants, loans, and technical assistance to those who wished to start or expand HMOs; and the inclusion of a mandatory HMO option in all forms of health insurance.

The second assumption was that new HMOs will be as effective as existing prototypes in reducing hospitalization, and in allocating critical resources such as primary physicians and hospital beds more efficiently. Some opponents argued that existing organizations are marginal forms of care, staffed by atypical doctors, and serving healthy employed groups whose medical needs are not comparable to those of the general population. Proponents countered that neither the organizations nor their enrollees are atypical, and that, when allowance is made for population differences, the evidence shows that the efficiency of existing HMOs is significantly greater than that of the conventional practice sector.[10] Since new HMOs would embody the same incentives and operational principles as the prototypes, it seemed reasonable to assume that they would perform with comparable efficiency.

The third assumption was that, as HMOs become more numerous, competition will increase and have a positive effect on the performance of both fee-for-service providers and HMOs themselves. Unlike the previous assumptions there was little direct evidence to support this belief. The prospect of competition from Kaiser is believed to have spurred the founding of the nation's first risk-sharing medical society foundation plans in California and Oregon (see below, p. 61), and Kaiser, in turn, acknowledges that its pricing policies are based in part on the rates charged by "the Blues" and indemnity insurance companies. However, apart from these isolated and indirect suggestions of its validity, the basis for this assumption lay primarily in economic theory and principles. At present, physicians and other health professionals exercise nearly total dominance over the health industry's structure, its practice patterns, the prices of services, and the regulatory mechanisms that govern provider performance.[11] Market forces, such as competition and informed consumer choice, are thought to have little impact. However, it was assumed that, if market forces could be set in motion, they would provide an effective check on inflation, uneven quality, maldistribution, and the provision of unnecessary services.

The final assumption was the most tenuous of all because contingent on the realization of the first three. It was assumed that—if new HMOs form and perform like the operating prototypes, and if the competition they engender has a favorable effect on the performance of all providers—then the need for more government planning and regulation will be greatly reduced and political demands for expanded public control will cease. This assumption captures the essence of the HMO strategy, which is aimed at promoting a largely self-governing health industry in which provider behavior is motivated by internal incentives to be responsive to consumer demands. The belief that the drive for public regulation was based fundamentally on performance grounds rather than ideological principles about the proper ethical position of those who serve the sick, seemed to support this assumption. While its logic is consistent with the premises on which it is based, the assumption's validity obviously hinges on whether the events foreseen in the previous assumptions unfold as predicted.

As these assumptions suggest, the transition to a health system in which market influences operate to bring provider performance more in line with the public interest was expected to take time. It was also recognized that whether the transition occurred at all hinged on the willingness of decision makers to take the necessary steps to implement change, and refrain from imposing irrevocable regulatory controls during the change-over period.

RECENT DEVELOPMENTS IN THE HEALTH INDUSTRY

Despite widespread initial endorsement by government leaders, industry spokesmen, and other public leaders,[12] formal action to implement the HMO strategy has been slow in coming. Moreover, the debate surrounding the HMO enabling bill and related health matters makes it clear that the issue of more regulation versus the incentives approach to solving our health delivery problems is far from resolved.

On the federal level, the HMO concept enjoys strong bipartisan approval, but congressional deliberation over enabling measures has been cautious and thoughtful. After three years of discussion and debate, the HMO Enabling Act became Public Law 93-222 on December 29, 1973. Congressional action to amend the Social Security Act to allow Medicare beneficiaries to enroll in HMOs was less drawn out, but the reimbursement provisions of the Medicare "HMO option" represent an approach that might be described as "cost-plus with a ceiling." It also contains numerous regulatory features that are counter to the intent of the HMO concept, and more in keeping with the notion of continued public regulation and control.

Meanwhile, unexpectedly strong support has developed in Congress and among state government leaders and others for proposals aimed at converting the health industry into a state-regulated public utility.[13] To many, a public regulatory agency, empowered to regulate the rates charged by health providers, the territories they serve, and the quality of the services they provide, offers the most immediate and decisive way to curtail inflation and improve the quality and availability of health services. Hence, the recent passage of the HMO Enabling Act should not be interpreted to mean that Congress has decided to pursue the incentive approach in preference to a public utility form of regulation.

The executive branch has also wavered in its support of the HMO strategy. Following its initial endorsement and its early attempts to assist the formation of new HMOs, the administration has gradually drawn back from an all out commitment to this approach. This toning down of support has been due in part to the mobilization of HMO opponents and their success in pressuring the administration to change its original position. But it is also due to a loss of institutional memory in the face of numerous personnel changes, and to the ever present political obsession to do something new this year. While this does not necessarily signal a shift toward the regulatory approach, some influential members of the administration doubt the validity of the HMO approach and favor the use of continuing and permanent regulatory controls.

Despite this mixed response by government bodies and professional groups and the lack of a clear-cut legal climate for implementing the HMO strategy, a quiet revolution is going on in the health industry that is only beginning to attract public notice. What follows is a summary of a few of the developments that have taken place over the past three years, in terms of their import for the original assumptions of the HMO strategy.

The Health Industry Can Be Restructured

Are providers responding to federal initiatives by forming HMOs as it was assumed they would? The response to the HMO idea to date has undoubtedly exceeded anyone's earlier expectations. Tangible evidence supporting that conclusion is now available in the form of findings from a nationwide survey that InterStudy is conducting to identify all operating HMOs and those that are either in the process of formation or under active study.[14] Preliminary data indicate the extent and magnitude of HMO formation and growth. As of January 1974—

- There are at least 172 operating HMOs in 33 states and the District of Columbia (Table 1), compared with 25 prototype organizations operating in 12 states in January, 1970.
- At least 152 additional HMOs are in the process of formation, and another 125 prospective sponsoring groups are actively studying the possibility of forming HMOs, in all but 3 of the 50 states.
- Since January, 1970, enrollment in HMOs is conservatively estimated to have increased by about 635,000; new HMOs have enrolled 428,000 subscribers, while enrollment in existing organizations has increased by 207,000.[15]

InterStudy's survey is also examining the socioeconomic and legal factors associated with HMO formation, by comparing selected variables in states with one or more HMOs with the same variables in non-HMO states. Findings show that new HMOs tend to behave like other economic entities, and thus have gravitated first to areas with the most favorable markets and the fewest legal barriers. For example, HMOs are forming in states with higher average family incomes, larger and more highly urbanized populations, more physicians per capita, higher hospital daily costs, larger per capita expenditures for medical care, and more multispecialty group practices. HMO states also have fewer hospital beds and use hospital services less frequently than non-HMO states. Two legal variables were found to be strongly related to the absence of HMOs: Non-HMO states typically have strict physician control and open panel requirements governing the operation of health plans.

These data document the recent rapid growth of HMOs and provide substantiation for the assumption that HMOs would form in large numbers, given the provision of appropriate incentives. Since market considerations and local legal climates are prime determinants for HMO development, the provisions of Public Law 93-222 (the HMO Act), which are aimed at enhancing the market (i.e., by requiring employee health plans to include the option of HMO membership) and eliminating restrictive state laws (i.e., by federal pre-emption), are "right on target," and can be expected to accelerate HMO growth even further. It should be pointed out, however, that without some equalization of consumer purchasing power, it is unrealistic to expect that health services can be ideally distributed, or that a majority of the U.S. population will be able to enroll in HMOs.

TABLE 1 HMOs by State, January, 1974

	No. HMOs in Operation	HMOs in Formation or Planning	
		Formation	Planning
Alabama	2		1
Alaska		2	
Arizona	6		2
Arkansas			1
California	65	29	40
Colorado	2	4	2
Connecticut	2	2	3
Delaware		1	1
District of Columbia	3	3	1
Florida	3	12	7
Georgia		2	
Hawaii	6		2
Idaho			
Illinois	14	4	5
Indiana	1	2	1
Iowa	1	1	
Kansas	1	2	1
Kentucky	2	3	2
Louisiana		1	1
Maine	2	1	
Maryland	6	6	2
Massachusetts	3	5	2
Michigan	5	6	
Minnesota	7	4	5
Mississippi		1	1
Missouri	4	1	4
Montana			
Nebraska		1	1
Nevada	1	2	1
New Hampshire	1		1
New Jersey	2	7	
New Mexico	2	1	
New York	7	10	6
North Carolina	1	2	1
North Dakota		1	1
Ohio	2	7	2
Oklahoma		1	1
Oregon	3	1	1
Pennsylvania	3	11	3
Rhode Island	2	1	1
South Carolina	1	2	
South Dakota			
Tennessee		1	3
Texas	1	2	2
Utah		3	
Vermont		1	
Virginia		2	2
Washington	3	1	7
West Virginia	2		7
Wisconsin	6	2	1
Wyoming		1	
TOTAL	172	152	125

New HMOs Will Be As Effective As the Prototypes

What about the second assumption? Are new HMOs reducing hospitalization and allocating their resources more efficiently, like the established prototypes? While it is still rather early to evaluate their performance generally, some new HMOs are performing much more efficiently than the fee-for-service sector, despite the fact that they are staffed by physicians previously engaged exclusively in fee-for-service practice. The three HMOs described below illustrate what is taking place.

The MedCenter Health Plan was developed by an existing 75-man multispecialty group practice located in St. Louis Park, a Minneapolis suburb. It became operational about one year ago and now enrolls about 5000 subscribers. Table 2 summarizes MedCenter's first-year experience in terms of selected performance indicators, and compares that experience with comparable statewide data. While an attempt has been made to adjust the data for differences in age and employment status in the two groups, the adjustment process was admittedly crude and, thus, the data should be interpreted accordingly. Nevertheless, a more precise statistical analysis would not substantially alter the large differences in performance indicated in the table. As shown, insured Minnesotans who obtain health services from conventional sources use more than 2½ times as many hospital days as MedCenter enrollees, and require 3 times as many hospital beds. This marked difference in MedCenter's use of costly hospital services is the result of its lower admission rate and average length of stay, both of which are approximately half as large as those of the fee-for-service sector in Minnesota. By making more extensive use of ambulatory services, and by controlling the use of hospital services, MedCenter, like its more established HMO forebears, is already demonstrating that, given the appropriate incentives, it can provide quality health services more efficiently and economically than conventional practitioners.

One of the first of the new group of HMOs to begin operation is the Greater Marshfield Community Health Plan (GMCHP), which began

TABLE 2 MedCenter Performance vs. Performance Statewide (first-year)

Indicators of Performance	MedCenter Health Plan	State of Minnesota
Hospital admissions/1000 pop.	78	168
Average length of stay (days)	4.8	8.7
Hospital days/1000 pop.	475	1220
Hospital beds/1000 pop.	1.9	5.7

doing business in April, 1971. Like MedCenter, the GMCHP was developed by a highly respected 118-member fee-for-service multispecialty physician group, the Marshfield Clinic, located in a town of 15,000 in rural Wisconsin. The plan is managed and marketed through a cooperative arrangement with Wisconsin Blue Cross, which negotiates annual capitation contracts with the clinic and two local hospitals for medical and inpatient services. All participating entities share in savings realized through efficient operation. From its inception, enrollment in the Marshfield HMO has been genuinely open. In fact, plan representatives literally went door to door soliciting subscribers and enrolled about half of the town's population during the first three months of the Plan's existence. Membership has increased steadily and currently is about 18,000.

One reason for this continued growth has been that unique working affiliations have been developed with 15 primary physicians in small towns surrounding Marshfield. These solo and small group physicians continue to work out of their own office, and are paid on a fee-for-service basis plus an annual incentive bonus for efficient practice. This branching arrangement enables the Marshfield HMO to disperse its points of entry and expand its service area, a feature that is especially valuable to residents of a somewhat sparsely populated rural area, and one which resembles the idealized "planetary" model that we health planners talk about but rarely produce.

Table 3 compares the performance of the Marshfield HMO with that of Wisconsin practitioners who employ conventional delivery and payment modes. (Like the MedCenter data, an attempt has been made to adjust for differences in age and employment status in the two population groups, but the Wisconsin data also are admittedly error-prone.) Probably because of its open enrollment, Marshfield's utilization rates are proportionately somewhat higher than those of the MedCenter HMO, but they are substantially lower than those of Wisconsin's fee-for-service sector. GMCHP enrollees use less than half as many hospital days as insured Wisconsin residents in general.

The third example is the Physicians Association of Clackamus County,

TABLE 3 GMCHP Performance vs. Performance Statewide

Indicators of Performance	Marshfield GMCHP	State of Wisconsin
Hospital admissions/1000 pop.	97	158
Average length of stay (days)	5.7	8.4
Hospital days/1000 pop.	549	1165
Hospital beds/1000 pop.	2.0	5.0

Oregon (PACC), which was established by the county medical society more than 30 years ago to offer prepaid medical service plans to interested groups. Its member physicians agreed to absorb all underwriting losses themselves without the involvement of third parties. To maintain effective control against unnecessary services and unjustified costs, PACC has developed elaborate claims–utilization review mechanisms to evaluate the fees and charges of each participating physician against county-wide, monthly cost-per-case averages.

In 1970, PACC began marketing an HMO health plan, called the "Protective Circle Plan," which provides comprehensive health services to about 6000 enrollees. Subscribers may obtain medical services from any of the 151 participating physicians, who practice in their own offices throughout the service area. Thirteen hospitals, 37 pharmacies, 7 medical laboratories, 17 optometrists, and 2 physical therapy centers also participate in the plan. Like physician participants, they too are "at risk" for a proportionate share of any operating losses the plan may incur. All professional and institutional participants are reimbursed monthly at 80 percent of their allowed fees or charges, with the remaining income from subscriber premiums pooled to cover unforeseen expenses. Surpluses from this pooled reserve are distributed to the several participants annually to bring payments up to 100 percent of their allowed fees or charges, but participants are not permitted to bill subscribers for any unpaid balance.

PACC's 35 years of experience in cost-conscious health delivery have resulted in the superior performance of all its health plans. Even so, the cost of its HMO plan is 8–18 percent less than the cost of comparable benefits under its other medical services plans. Table 4 compares the performance of both types of PACC health plans with that of Oregon's fee-for-service sector. (Again, allowance has been made for population differences in the groups served.) The data show that PACC's regular plans compare favorably with many HMOs, and that its HMO plan is functioning even more efficiently.

TABLE 4 PACC Performance vs. Performance Statewide

	PACC		
Indicators of Performance	Protective Circle	Regular	State of Oregon
Hospital admissions/1000 pop.	103	117	144
Average length of stay (days)	3.9	4.6	6.8
Hospital days/1000 pop.	406	544	854
Hospital beds/1000 pop.	1.9	2.1	3.8

The Competitive Health Market Will Work

What about the third assumption? Is there any evidence that new HMOs are engendering competition with conventional practitioners, and, if so, is competition improving the performance of either or both?

In general, HMOs do not yet command a large enough segment of local markets to make their competitive influence felt, and thus it is too early to say whether this assumption will be fully borne out. However, in areas where HMOs are especially strong, there are some indications that the fee-for-service sector is at least beginning to take notice of their presence.

As already mentioned, the threat of competition from HMOs was a major motive in the formation of the risk-sharing medical society foundation plans that have developed in California and Oregon, programs incidentally on which the PSRO regulatory approach was based. Steinwald[16] writes:

> The first Foundation for Medical Care was established in 1954 in the San Joaquin Valley, California. Rumors of the expansion of the Kaiser Medical Foundation, a prepaid group practice, distressed Valley physicians who viewed closed panel practices as a threat to the solo practice of medicine. To counteract the spread of Kaiser, the San Joaquin Medical Society developed a program which would incorporate some of the attractive features of Kaiser with private medical practice. The result was a medical society sponsored prepaid health insurance plan in which physicians would be reimbursed on a fee-for-service basis.

In addition to the San Joaquin program, which clearly antedates the current movement, seven other foundation-based HMOs have formed in California in the past three years, and nine others are in the process of formation. Moreover, physicians who practice in mixed arrangements, where their time is divided between HMO patients and fee-for-service patients, report that their HMO practice habits are having an effect on the way they manage their fee-for-service patients as well.

A more obvious example of the impact of HMOs can be found in the current situation in Southern California, where strong competition has recently developed between new prepaid health plans (PHPs, as HMOs are called in California) and conventional practitioners.[17] Nowhere has the notion of using public money to reshape the health system been implemented more resolutely than in California. Interest in delivery system reform was aroused by sky-rocketing public expenditures for the state's Medi-Cal program, which was heading toward a potential deficit of $50 million. Since Medi-Cal is funded by a fixed annual appropriation, immediate action was essential. Rather than asking for a supplemental appropriation or cutting back on the number of eligible beneficiaries, the Department of Health Care Services decided on a different course. Physicians were ordered to hospitalize Medi-Cal patients only when it was absolutely necessary, and only after obtaining written authorization from the state. Subsequently, these "emergency" administration measures were written into law by the California Assembly, but were applied only to conventional fee-for-service doctors. PHPs, which had demonstrated that they used hospital services sparingly, and members of physician-sponsored admissions review groups, were explicitly exempt. By selectively applying this new rule, it was hoped that physicians would be encouraged to develop new forms of practice to free themselves of such odious control. At the same time, positive efforts were launched to foster the development of prepaid health plans and to encourage PHP enrollment by Medi-Cal patients.

This strategy has had a dramatic impact on California's health industry. In the past two years about 50 new PHPs have formed, which currently provide care for approximately 200,000 Medi-Cal patients; and more than twice as many prospective PHPs are being planned. Private physicians have been far from sanguine over these events, particularly in Southern California where most new PHPs are located. They complain that the new groups are deceiving Medi-Cal patients with aggressive enrollment practices and extravagant promises that they fail to make good. They also allege that some PHPs are skimping on services and/or delivering substandard care. In a few cases, court action has been initiated to restrain unscrupulous operators, and one county medical society is openly urging Medi-Cal patients to disenroll from PHPs and is providing them with assistance to do so. Interestingly, opposition to the new PHPs has the backing of a variety of organizations with varied political persuasions, including the labor union sponsored California Plan for Health Care Alternatives and several welfare rights groups.

Critics have called attention to several weaknesses in California's PHP program that could have given rise to abuses. For one thing, since the program focuses solely on the poor, PHPs deal with the most naïve of all health consumers, where the possibility of exploitation by unscrupulous operators is high. Further, new PHPs serve areas were the dearth of health services sharply limits the residents' opportunity to choose among alternative health providers. California has tried to introduce competition in such areas by granting franchises to more than one PHP, but consumer choice is still restricted. Finally, the California program failed to include safeguards against the entry of marginal, or "fast buck," operators, although steps are being taken to correct this shortcoming.

The lessons of the California experience have not been wasted. For one thing, they played a significant part in shaping the quality and grievance sections of the new federal law. Under the new act, would-be HMOs must commit themselves to establish stable, continuing programs, since the level of investment they are required to make in capital and start-up costs can only be recouped over a period of several years. Safeguards are also included to ensure that new HMOs serve a balanced patient mix, rather than serving just the old and the poor. California is taking steps to revise its PHP program to include these same safeguards, and has also begun to develop a very advanced and sophisticated quality assurance program.

Critics of the market approach point to the California situation as evidence of the dangers inherent in relying on competitive forces to control provider behavior. But proponents argue that the situation merely illustrates what the market is all about. They contend that the improvements that are now being implemented will mean that, in the long run, market forces will eliminate marginal operators and improve the performance of all providers.

If HMOs Succeed, The Need and Desire for Expanded Regulation Will Diminish

What about the last and most crucial assumption? Is there any indication that promising developments in the health industry are dampening the drive for stricter regulation? All of the "readable" signs seem to point in the opposite direction. The current political climate, coupled with the industry's continuing failure to develop and actively promote credible alternatives to regulation, are accelerating the pressure for more stringent controls.

Regulatory efforts at present are piecemeal, but as a next step the administration and others have pulled the pieces together through the vehicle of the national health insurance plans they have proposed, and through comprehensive planning and regulatory legislation that may be enacted to replace the expiring CHP, RMP, and Hill–Burton programs. In the past two years alone two major regulatory programs have been installed, beginning with price controls, which were first applied as a part of the administration's economic stabilization program. Moreover, while price controls have been relaxed in most other sectors of the economy, the indications are that they will not only be continued in the health industry for a long time to come, but that controls may be expanded to cover the quantity of services provided as well.[18]

The amendments to the Social Security Act, which created the Professional Standards Review Organizations and put teeth into hospital planning, also represent a major step toward more stringent public control over health providers. Responsibility for PSRO administration was vested in physicians themselves, but the threat is implicit that, should they fail to do the job, the federal government will take over. Thus, rather than attempting to intrinsically modify provider behavior through the use of incentives, Congress elected to publicly impose external controls.

To further complicate an already confusing situation, a number of positive and spontaneous market adjustments are taking place within the health industry that could have a corrective effect and reduce the need for external controls. For example, hospital managers are finding that, for a variety of reasons, it is becoming increasingly difficult to build new hospital beds. This is due in part to such factors as the tight money market, high interest rates, the possibility that HMOs and PSROs will decrease hospital use, and uncertainty about the rapidly changing regulatory climate. But it is also clear that hospitals are beginning to get the message that surplus beds beget excessive use, and therefore they are a major inflationary factor that must be resolved.

Similar self-correcting activities could help to bring medical specialty distributions into closer alignment with actual consumer needs. Like entrepreneurs in other sectors of the economy, physicians are capable of generating a demand for the services they provide. This ability, coupled with surpluses in certain specialty fields, is widely believed to result in the provision of unnecessary services that contribute to rising health costs. In surgery, where surpluses have been evident for some time, surgeons themselves are beginning to search for ways to limit the future supply of surgeons. Voluntary action such as this, taken by surplus specialty groups in their own professional interest, could moderate the specialty imbalance problem if they are allowed time to work themselves out. Otherwise, the growing concern over the shortage of primary and rural doctors in the face of surplus physicians in certain high-cost prestige specialties, will almost certainly give rise to a new form of public control, a health manpower regulatory agency, empowered to determine how many physicians are produced, the number of training slots available in various fields, and possibly where physicians will be allowed to practice.

These natural adjustments are not a prelude to utopia, but when taken together with the growth of HMOs and other major structural developments in the health industry, they should not be taken lightly. It would be ironic indeed if, in our haste to decisively resolve our health delivery problems, we should elect to impose external controls that not only prove unnecessary, but difficult to disengage once they are in place, and whose very existence is likely to foreclose the possibility that providers will continue to move toward a more competitive and self-regulating health system.

IS THE HMO STRATEGY ENOUGH?

Despite the rapid and promising changes taking place within the health industry, it is becoming clear that something more is needed to change the current political mood favoring more decisive action. Whatever impact the new HMO Enabling Act may have in accelerating these changes, it will still take time to make the transition to a system in which HMOs command a significant share of the health market. And it will take longer still for the effects of a competitive market to make themselves felt in the industry's overall performance. Since the urgency of finding solutions to current problems is not likely to allow the luxury of time, interim measures are needed that will quickly ameliorate our most urgent problems without imposing permanent regulatory controls. If such actions can be devised, it may yet be possible to buy the necessary time required for the improvements implicit in the market-oriented approach to fully evolve.

The proposals that follow are put forth with that objective in mind, although they are not the only measures that could be taken, nor are they necessarily the best. They arise out of two fundamental convictions: that it is better to make the health system work efficiently by using incentives to modify the behavior of patients and health providers than to seek this goal by imposing external controls; and that, if controls must be employed as a last resort (a circumstance that seems to exist at present), such measures should be consistent with the competitive incentives approach, be applied objectively and decisively, and be capable of being withdrawn at the earliest feasible moment without creating the need for permanent regulatory control.

Some of the suggestions outlined below will appeal, it is hoped, to those who advocate an incentive approach. But it is not likely that any of them will satisfy those who advocate public regulatory control on the ideological ground that matters as grave as health care cannot be left to the whims that govern individual consumers and providers in their marketplace decisions, especially when the provision of health services is heavily financed by public tax funds.

For many of us the paramount question is, How can our critical problems be solved without destroying the climate of voluntary change? Is it possible to devise credible proposals to meet this objective that can win the support of a large segment of the industry's major actors and be salable to political decision makers as well? Admittedly, these are formidable requirements and they can be met only by including measures that some will find unpalatable. But half-way measures are not likely to succeed in heading off the current drive for tighter regulatory control.

The suggestions offered below fall into three categories: (1) providing consumer information, (2) incentives to encourage greater hospital efficiency, and (3) continued support for competitive delivery systems.

Providing Consumer Information

These measures are aimed at correcting a major hindrance to effective competition: the consumer's lack of information about where to obtain needed health services, and how to assess the appropriateness, quality, and price of the services he receives.[19] Lack of such information obviously places consumers at the mercy of providers and creates a climate that is conducive to market dysfunction. Rather than trying to correct these defects by such stringent and uncertainly effective measures as franchising and permanent rate controls, a deliberate effort could be made to promote informed buying decisions by the consuming public. Three specific measures that might further this objective are the following:

1. *Publication of Consumer Guides.* Consumers and providers should be provided with up-to-date, easily understandable information, perhaps in the form of consumer guides, about alternative sources of health care available in their communities. These guides would include information on the prices and quality of local professional and hospital services, health insurance plans, prescription drugs, and so on.[20]
2. *Enactment of "Truth in Health Insurance" Legislation.* Legislation analogous to the Truth in Lending Act should be passed to require that health insurance policies be written in language that is easily understandable to the layman, and in a form that facilitates comparison of the costs and benefits offered by each health insurance policy. It might also require the inclusion of certain guaranteed rights for the insured, such as non-cancelability.
3. *Establishing a Health Education Program.* A systematic program of health education should be launched to provide consumers with information on good health practices, including how to avoid illness, how major diseases can be recognized and treated, what constitutes ideal health care, and so on. One possibility would be to follow the guidelines recently laid down by the President's Commission on Health Education.

Responsibility for the development and direction of this varied program of consumer information could be given to the CHP agencies, since they already have extensive knowledge of available health resources.

Incentives to Encourage Greater Hospital Efficiency

A second set of measures focuses explicitly on hospitals, since the hospital sector is acknowledged to be the most inflationary component of our health delivery system. While these measures are consistent with the competitive market incentives approach and would have an immediate and potentially large payoff in savings, they would not require the imposition of controls that could inhibit the entry of competing, less costly institutional arrangements, and have a powerful "tar baby" effect.[21]

1. *Changing Hospital Reimbursement.* A uniform hospital reimbursement system should be devised and installed that would shift payment away from existing cost reimbursement formulas to incentive arrangements that reward hospitals for providing quality services at reasonable cost. Present reimbursement practices favor some third parties, while discriminating against others. Moreover, cost reimbursement provides the incentive to add to, and embellish, hospital services, rather than encouraging efficient management. Without doubt, much of the drive for rate regulation is motivated by this desire to reimburse hospitals on a sound and rational basis.

2. *Revising the Hill–Burton Program.* The objectives of the Hill–Burton program should be revised from subsidizing the construction of new hospital beds, to funding and encouraging modernization and capital facilities that increase productivity.

3. *Taking Hospital Beds Out of Production.* It is widely agreed that a surplus of hospital beds exists, and that this surplus is a major contributor to excessive hospital use. To counter this problem some have proposed an across-the-board freeze on increased hospital capacity, and the elimination of tax deductions for charitable contributions for this purpose. However, solving the surplus hospital bed problem will require more than inhibiting the construction of new beds. Ways must also be found to take surplus beds out of production. Major trends are under way that point inexorably toward decreased hospital use. One is the growth of HMOs, which use only about half as many beds as are presently available. Another is the increasingly effective application of preadmission and utilization review procedures, which have already demonstrated their ability to reduce hospitalization. Hence, it is vital that

ways be found to reduce our present hospital bed supply. One way is by establishing a "bed bank" program, whereby financial assistance could be provided to conscientious hospitals with empty beds due to increased efficiency. Such funds could be used to encourage hospitals to convert unused beds into ambulatory care clinics, doctor's offices, and other needed and innovative purposes.

Continued Support for Competitive Delivery Systems

The federal government should continue to encourage the development of competing innovative forms of health delivery that demonstrate the ability to provide quality services at lower cost, as it has done in the case of HMOs. The passage of the HMO Enabling Act now seems to assure that HMOs will get a fair market test. But if other health delivery arrangements are advanced that show promise of enhancing the health market, similar assistance should be provided to assure a fair test of their viability. It would be better still to actively promote such arrangements by an organized program of health system development. One way this could be done is by reshaping the objectives of the Regional Medical Program around this goal, since many are determined to keep RMP alive in some form.

Finally, it should be understood that these suggestions are not put forth as a comprehensive or permanent health care program, but as a set of short-term expedient measures designed to achieve a particular purpose. For example, a vigorous medical market obviously requires that health insurance coverage be extended to all who need care but cannot afford it. Yet, this vital issue has not been discussed. It is also important that the health industry begin to shift to an outcomes-oriented quality assurance system to replace the present system of input and process measures that have little relationship to the quality of the services produced.[22] But the quality issue, too, has been omitted in this paper. (Incidentally, one of the important side benefits of the HMO Enabling Act is that it further emphasizes, and provides needed financial support for, the development of a better quality assurance system.) The omission of these crucial issues is not meant to diminish their importance, but to underscore the importance of continuing to give top priority to the task of restructuring the health delivery system. Only then can we reasonably expect that advanced quality assurance systems and noninflationary financing arrangements will work in the way we intend them to work.

ACKNOWLEDGMENT

The author is grateful for the collaborative work on this paper by Earl J. Hoagberg, research associate, InterStudy.

REFERENCES AND NOTES

1. As originally set forth, the HMO strategy proposed "a series of steps over a 5–10-year period in which the federal government would: (1) adopt the health maintenance strategy and call upon both private enterprise and public agencies to join the health industry in implementing the national objective of health maintenance; (2) provide incentives for creation of health maintenance organizations; (3) foster the elimination of any legal barriers which may block creation of such organizations; (4) begin purchasing services under Medicare, Medicaid, and other federal reimbursement programs by health maintenance contracts rather than by the present method of paying for individual medical services; (5) build into these contracts a sufficient return to support necessary investments in manpower, facilities, and health services research by the contracting health maintenance organizations; (6) review its activities in the health field to determine how they currently contribute to, or frustrate, the health maintenance strategy, and initiate necessary modifications to support it." (See Ellwood PM, Jr et al.: Health maintenance strategy, Med Care IX(3):291–298, 1971.)
2. Medicare and Medicaid–Problems, Issues, and Alternatives (Report of the Staff to the Committee on Finance, U.S. Senate), February 9, 1970.
3. See Report of the Task Force on Medicaid and Related Programs. U.S. Department of Health, Education, and Welfare. Washington, D.C., U.S. Government Printing Office, June, 1970.
4. Cf. Cutting C: Historical development and operating concepts, Chapter 2, in The Kaiser-Permanente Medical Care Program–A Symposium. Edited by A Somers. New York, The Commonwealth Fund, 1971. See page 19.
5. Many of the specific concerns expressed by various groups and individuals during the recent congressional hearings on the HMO enabling bill are summarized by J Iglehart in Health report: House panel moves toward compromise HMO plan despite strong opposition, Natl J (May 6, 1972), p 780.
6. In a press release on March 25, 1970, HEW Secretary Robert H. Finch said: ". . . we hope to accelerate the coming of a new era of diversity and competition for health care in the U.S., based on informed consumer choices and private incentives that operate within the framework of government safeguards. . . . We will not prescribe the form of a health maintenance organization but we will be concerned about the result it produces, much as we are concerned that those selling cars to the Federal government produce a quality product. Under such contracts [with HMOs] we will not pay separately for a specific surgical procedure, or a doctor's visit, any more than we pay separately for the essential parts of a car. We will be interested in delivery of an entire product, a guaranteed package of health benefits of high quality, and assurances that the organization can supply that product. The contract will

provide a set price per person per year. Savings through efficiencies consistent with quality care will go to the organization and to the consumer, and the organization will assume the risk of any losses."

7. One obvious example is the growth of group practice. In 1931, 99 percent of all private practitioners were in solo practice, but by 1969, nearly 18 percent of all practicing doctors were members of groups. (Cf. Profile of Medical Practice. Chicago, American Medical Association, 1971. See page 42.)
8. In a 1971 survey, Mechanic found that 51 percent of the 2200 primary doctors he surveyed expressed either "strong" or "moderate" approval of "prepaid group practice such as Kaiser-Permanente or the Health Insurance Plan of New York." (See Mechanic D: General medical practice: Some comparisons between the work of primary care physicians in the U.S. and England and Wales, Med Care X(5), 1972.) A more recent AMA survey of U.S. physicians in general indicates that 30 percent of the AMA members in the sample and 47 percent of the non-members "expressed a preference for some type of prepaid capitation practice over fee-for-service practice." (See Questions Physicians Are Asking About HMOs and the Answers. Washington, D.C., Department of Health, Education, and Welfare, December 1972.)
9. See Holley R, Carlson RJ: The Legal Context for the Development of Health Maintenance Organizations. Minneapolis, InterStudy, 1971.
10. One of the most comprehensive summaries of comparative performance data on prepaid group practice plans and conventional providers is that of Avedis Donabedian. See An evaluation of prepaid group practice, Inquiry VI (3), 1969. The tables shown below are indicative of the superior performance of one "HMO prototype" over fee-for-service providers:

Per Capita Expenditures: Medical Care Nationwide vs. Kaiser Plan in California

	Expenditures ($)		
	1960	1965	1968
All U.S.			
Hospital care	49.35	68.47	101.73
Physicians' services	31.02	44.28	54.79
TOTAL	80.37	112.75	156.52
Kaiser's California Regions			
Hospital care	18.97	21.11	28.56
Physicians' services	39.22	47.84	63.84
TOTAL	58.19	68.95	92.40

SOURCE: Social Security Bulletin, Jan 1970; and Report of National Advisory Commission on Health Manpower, Nov 1967. Kaiser disputes the figures of the commission report.

Member Utilization: Kaiser Plan vs. Two Other U.S. Plans

	Hospital Days per 1,000 Persons		
Year	Blue Cross[a]	Indemnity[b] (Aetna)	Kaiser[c]
1962	1,111	842	544
1963	1,146	896	493
1964	1,159	1,020	504
1965	1,194	1,102	457
1966	1,195	852[d]	460
1967	954	799[d]	441
1968	901	815[d]	497
1969	892	–	494
1970	894	–	480[e]

SOURCE: Modern Hospital, Blue Cross Assoc., Aetna Life & Casualty, Kaiser Foundation, and U.S. Civil Service Commission.
[a]Fiscal year basis.
[b]Selected federal high option plans.
[c]Calendar year basis.
[d]Average Aetna groups.
[e]Estimate.

11. For example, licensing boards in most states typically are composed of representatives from the regulated profession, who are selected by each governor upon recommendation of the appropriate professional society. About half of the licensure laws require all members of the board to be licensed practitioners. (See State Licensing of Health Occupations, Public Health Serv Publ No. 1758, Washington, D.C., U.S. Government Printing Office, 1967.) Moreover, even though CHP agencies are required to have a majority of consumers, that slender majority is often eroded through lack of attendance on the part of consumer representatives, or by their lack of understanding of the many issues under discussion. Thus, as a practical matter, many CHP agencies are effectively dominated by providers who are both "committee wise" and generally more knowledgeable about the issues at stake. (See also Footnote 22, page 85, in Ellwood PM, Jr et al.: Assuring the Quality of Health Care. Minneapolis, InterStudy, 1973.)
12. The success of the HMO strategy, in large part, is the result of the endorsements of President Nixon and HEW Secretaries Robert Finch and Elliot Richardson, as well as of such leaders of the Democratic party as Senator Edward M. Kennedy and Congressmen Paul Rogers and William R. Roy. Backing by leaders such as these and other influential persons undoubtedly helped to stimulate the formation of HMOs, and the rapid HMO enrollment that is going on today.
13. For example, HR 12053, referred to the Interstate and Foreign Commerce Committee on December 20, 1973, calls for amending the PHS Act to assure the development of a national health policy, and to create effective state regulatory programs and areawide health planning programs.
14. See Schlenker R et al.: Socioeconomic and Legal Factors Associated with HMO presence: An Examination of State Data. Minneapolis, InterStudy, October 1973. For purposes of this survey, an HMO was defined as "an organization which accepts contractual responsibility to assure the delivery of a stated

range of health services, including at least ambulatory and in-hospital physician services and hospital care to a voluntarily enrolled population, in exchange for an advance capitation payment."

15. Based on replies to InterStudy's survey, we estimate that enrollment in HMOs that began operation after January, 1970, now totals approximately 428,000; HMOs established prior to January, 1970, have increased their enrollment by approximately 207,000 during the same period.
16. Steinwald C: An Introduction to Foundations for Medical Care. Chicago, Blue Cross Association, September 1971. See page 6.
17. For a description of the Southern California situation, see State medicine conservative style–Still a hassle, Med Econ (Sept 3, 1973), pp 171*ff*.
18. New Phase IV regulations, recently put into effect by the Cost of Living Council, are designed explicitly to encourage reductions in hospital admissions. Hospitals with decreases in admissions will be allowed to increase their charges to cover the increased costs of each admission, plus additional increases to cover fixed costs resulting from decreased admission rates. Those with increased admission rates will be limited to increases in charges to pay *only* for the costs connected with each additional admission. Thus, in larger hospitals, allowable increases in charges will range from about 17 percent in hospitals that have decreased admissions by 10 percent, to 3 percent in those that have increased admissions by 10 percent.
19. Currently, "ethical" restrictions on advertising, soliciting patients, competitive pricing, etc., imposed by licensure provisions and by various professional associations, prohibit providers from publishing information that might aid consumers in selecting sources of health care. (For example, see Principles of Medical Ethics, Section V. Chicago, American Medical Association, 1957).
20. Some groups such as the labor union-sponsored California Program for Health Care Alternatives, are already attempting to provide their members with information on alternative sources of care. The Pennsylvania Insurance Department, headed by Herbert S. Dennenberg, published a "Shopper's Guide to Hospitals in the Philadelphia Area," in November 1971, which included comparative average daily costs of 101 Philadelphia area hospitals. The guide was reprinted in 1972 along with a "Shopper's Guide to Surgery" and shopper's guides to Pennsylvania's auto insurance, life insurance, and term life insurance. Nader's organization is distributing a consumer-oriented "physician directory" in Prince Georges County, Maryland, which it expects will serve as the prototype for similar directories in other areas. In a related action, the Consumers Union recently sued the Veterans Administration seeking release of information to consumers on comparative performance of various hearing aids.
21. Experience in other regulated industries suggests that the domain of regulation tends to continually expand in order to plug the gaps in the existing regulatory structure. McKie has termed this phenomenon the "tar baby effect." See McKie JW: Regulation and the free market: The problem of boundaries, Bell J Econ Manage Sci 1(1):9, 1970.
22. For a more detailed discussion of the quality assurance problem and how quality assessment can be shifted to an outcome-oriented system, see Ellwood PM, Jr et al.: *op. cit.* (ref 11).

III

Regulation of Supply in Health Care

Two major resources of health care are the hospitals and other institutions that serve as loci for services, and the manpower required to perform those services. In this section, Clark C. Havighurst reviews the certification-of-need laws that control hospital construction in many states, and the conditions that gave rise to the laws; he concludes that they are designed "to preserve the very financing mechanisms that create the problems to which they are addressed." Alonzo Yerby traces the development of manpower regulation and reviews the present situation in which so many new regulatory proposals are being advanced.

Panelists who discussed these papers were Claude Castonguay, actuary and former Minister of the Department of Social Affairs, Province of Quebec; Judith Lave, Ph.D., associate professor of Economics and Urban Processes, Carnegie–Mellon University; Robert Sigmond, executive vice president, Albert Einstein Medical Center, Philadelphia; and Anne R. Somers, associate professor, Department of Community Medicine, New Jersey–Rutgers Medical School.

CLARK C. HAVIGHURST, J.D.
Professor of Law, Duke University Law School

Regulation of Health Institutions

Whenever the possibility is raised that comprehensive regulation may not be the best means of dealing with the central problems of the health care system, some representatives of the hospital sector are apt to challenge the relevance of the question. The argument runs, in Anne Somers' words,[1] as follows:

> "[H] ow to regulate" questions have, for all practical purposes, displaced the "should we regulate" questions of the past. Some latter-day Adam Smiths advocate that the health care industry be made over in the image of a theoretical free-market economy. But such Utopian model-building, intellectually stimulating as it may be, has little relevance to an industry wherein two-fifths of total expenditures already come from government sources, and two-thirds of . . . the personal health care bill is paid through third parties. . . .
>
> Perhaps even more decisive is the fact that—whether we like it or not, whether good or bad—the health care industry, especially the hospital component, is already extensively controlled by both Federal and state governments. Few, if any, other industries have been subjected to so much piecemeal and uncoordinated regulation. Hardly any aspect of hospital operation—from the width of corridors and the number of fire extinguishers to the method of cost finding and accounting, and the overtime pay of the orderly—escapes the scrutiny of some public official.
>
> The prospect of repealing or rolling back this enormous body of statutory and administrative regulation is highly unrealistic.

Reprinted, with permission, from Hospitals 48(12):65–71, 1974.

The high quotient of truth in these observations suggests the need to formulate the issue more precisely.

It would indeed be quixotic to argue for eliminating all regulation in the health care world and for reposing trust only in the "invisible hand." It is possible, however, to distinguish comprehensive economic regulation, of the kind employed in public utility and transportation fields, from narrower kinds of regulation directed toward protecting the public's health and safety. There is also an essential difference between regulation that improves the functioning of a marketplace by removing distorting influences and correcting incentives and regulation that displaces the market altogether, substituting centralized decisions for a multiplicity of private decisions made under the constraints of external circumstances. The health care system is only beginning to experiment with those kinds of regulation that go beyond protecting public health and safety and that directly govern price, investment, and market entry. While regulation in the hospital world is indeed extensive, it is not yet universally true (now that the jerry-built and temporary Economic Stabilization Program has expired) that the price of hospital services is strictly controlled by government or that fully competent providers can be excluded from the health care marketplace solely on grounds of "public convenience and necessity."

It must be recognized that there has been considerable momentum, at both state and federal levels, in the direction of strengthening economic regulation of health care. Nevertheless, it is debatable whether we have reached the point of declaring comprehensive regulation to be inevitable and its appropriateness worthy of only academic discussion. Indeed, recent months have seen a growing awareness of the potential shortcomings of regulatory solutions and a consequent greater willingness to consider whether regulatory initiatives may not be so unpromising as to warrant a re-examination of market-oriented alternatives. Since choices are to be made in any event between imperfect solutions, our objective must be to examine relative imperfections—both strengths and weaknesses—and the prospects for improving the functioning of either system. This is fundamentally a pragmatic, not an ideological, undertaking. One step involves extensive exploration of the performance of regulators in other industry settings and careful evaluation of the analogies and lessons that might be drawn from those other regulatory experiences. In an article published in the *Virginia Law Review,*[2] I attempted such an evaluation. For the most part, this article summarizes the conclusions reached, with more deliberation, in that article.

Not only those individuals whom Anne Somers might class as "latter-day Adam Smiths" are skeptical about regulation in general. Surprising as it may seem, disenchantment with regulation is increasingly widespread among persons who cannot be so lightly dismissed. Thus, Ralph Nader[3] himself has been in the forefront of the effort to expose regulation's shortcomings, and in an article that he co-authored the arguments marshalled against regulation are pretty much those emphasized here. Unfortunately, the emerging sophistication about regulation's shortcomings has not yet penetrated the hospital sector, which up to now has shown signs of imposing excessive trust in the regulatory mechanisms available to government. It would be a positive first step if the health care system could accept Nader's formulation of the problem of developing regulatory policy: "At best, regulation is a negative process, occasionally enjoining bad behavior but rarely compelling good. Hence, our general . . . policy should encourage competition in our economy by minimizing regulation except where clearly necessary."[4] Naturally, reasonable minds will differ as to when regulation is "clearly necessary," but this formulation at least directs attention to the proper questions and avoids the trap of the self-fulfilling prophecy that more regulation is inevitable.

ENTRY AND INVESTMENT CONTROLS

Most critics of regulation reserve their greatest antipathy for controls on new entry into regulated markets. Surprisingly, the theoretical arguments for legally restricting entry into public utility and transportation industries are quite weak, and it is therefore easy to argue that entry controls were adopted primarily in the interest of the regulated firms themselves, perhaps as a quid pro quo for their accepting rate regulation and certain "public" responsibilities. Interestingly, the theoretical arguments for entry controls in the hospital sector through so-called certification-of-need laws are substantially more persuasive than the arguments for controlling entry into most other regulated industries. The arguments originate, of course, in the system of third-party payment and the control that providers apparently exert over demand for health services. These factors, and others, distort the incentives surrounding decisions on hospital investment. Because hospitals do not face an appreciable risk that creation of excess industry capacity will result in depressed (below-cost) prices, too many hospital beds are likely to be built. The costs of erroneous investment decisions are externalized—that is, borne in large part by the public through third-party payment mechanisms. The hospital market therefore invites over-investment by growth-conscious managers, whereas in other industries growth is deterred in all cases except where shortages exist or significant efficiency gains are expected.

Whatever the merits of certification-of-need laws and despite strong arguments for them, it is important to recognize that they are an attempt to deal with just one symptom of the larger problem of third-party payment. Far from addressing root causes, these laws contemplate the continued predominance of those financing mechanisms that encourage inefficiency by both guaranteeing recovery of providers' costs and externalizing the costs of physicians' and patients' consumption decisions. Not surprisingly, then, proponents of certification-of-need laws are generally found among those groups least willing to see fundamental changes in the way health services are financed. Therefore it is fair to regard certification-of-need laws as conservative measures, designed to preserve the very financing mechanisms that create the problems to which they are addressed.

A comparison of the rationale underlying certification of need with the enacted laws leads quickly to the conclusion that there is no theoretical justification for extending certification-of-need laws to cover facilities other than hospitals. Specifically, coverage of nursing homes and similar institutions is unwarranted because competition would serve consumers considerably better here than in the case of hospitals: A wider range of choice would always be presented, and, unlike marginal hospitals, the poorer homes could be expected to close their doors if consumers would not support them. Moreover, the important subjective element in the quality of nursing home care further strengthens the case for according greater scope to consumer choice—with major efforts devoted to improving opportunities for its informed exercise through improved information and the activities of social workers, ombudsmen, and patient advocates.

Perhaps the greatest potential for serious harm from certification-of-need requirements results from coverage of ambulatory care facilities, as provided for in the majority of the 23 states having such laws. Because ambulatory care is not regularly paid for on a cost-reimbursement basis, is not particularly the province of not-for-profit providers, and has not been characterized by overcapacity, its coverage by these laws is not easily justified. Of course, a persuasive case can be made for regulating the location of all physicians' offices on the basis of physicians' control of demand for their own as well as hospital services, but no state has yet had the courage to attempt to regulate entry by any but institutional providers, including HMOs, surgicenters, and some group practices.

The argument for controlling such ambulatory care facilities has to be based, not on their perverse behavior, but on the expectation that substitution of cheaper ambulatory care for inpatient care will leave empty hospital beds, which it is claimed will attract new patients and raise health care costs overall. This logic, founded on the so-called "Roemer effect," provides special bait for a classic regulatory trap, since one of the most nearly universal characteristics of regulators, even when they do not have the benefit of this added argument, is to retard changes that are threatening to the regulated interests. Regulation of ambulatory facilities, as provided for in the American Hospital Association's (AHA's) model certification-of-need bill, could be expected to inhibit the substitution of outpatient for inpatient care, with high, though incalculable, costs to the public.

AGENCY BEHAVIOR

The behavior of certification-of-need agencies is difficult to examine directly because of limited experience, poor data, and the unreliability of anecdotal evidence. But evaluation is possible using impressionistic evidence to confirm or to dispute the strength of the analogy to regulatory agencies charged with similar responsibility in other industries. In my article,[2] I employ a number of behavioral hypotheses derived from the experience of other agencies as interpreted by numerous scholars. Lengthy discussion yields a number of points suggesting that regulators of the health care system will do no better in the long run than regulators in other areas have done, giving the public substantially less than it deserves in the way of cost control. The circumstances giving rise to my doubts are as follows:

1. the political influence of the hospital industry in the health planning and certification-of-need process;
2. the lack of political pressure to do more than slow down the rate of cost increases—which means that political processes can at best merely stabilize the percentage of GNP devoted to health care, even though a substantial fraction of those billions might be better spent by society on other things;
3. the general implicit belief in the value of more and better health services of all kinds so long as obvious duplication is avoided, a belief that is shared not only by providers and health planners but also by so-called consumers who may be involved in the regulatory process but who will have no occasion to count directly the costs of new or improved services;
4. the actual and potential opportunities for using "internal subsidies"—funds generated by charging monopoly prices for certain popular

services—to provide other services that would not be purchased if priced at cost;

5. the orientation of health planners and regulators, not to planning of a technocratic variety, but to incremental change based on consensual processes and political bargaining; and

6. the difficulty of reconciling the need for a substantial contraction in the hospital industry with regulators' naturally protective attitude toward the regulated firms' investments and revenues.

All of these factors seem inherent in the regulatory process in health care and not subject to significant amelioration by any organizational improvements that would be feasible in any foreseeable political environment.

If one looks for factors in the health world that might offset the perverse regulatory tendencies stemming from the enumerated circumstances, there are few hopeful signs. While consumer involvement is sometimes thought of as a solution, the previously cited circumstances reveal reasons why this is a vain hope. Indeed, I sense that, while perhaps useful in altering some priorities, consumer involvement is primarily a device for making consumers share the responsibility for runaway inflation. I seriously doubt that it can be expected to end inflation or to force a reduction in the claims that health care providers make on the public pocketbook.

Some may see health planning as setting the health world apart for purposes of predicting regulatory behavior. But planning, if carefully examined, turns out to be largely a euphemism for "politics as usual," with possibly a slightly greater input from the consumer side. Far from upsetting the analogy, experience with health planning generally confirms expectations drawn from other regulatory experience.

In summary, there is no reason to think regulation in the health sector will be exempt from the faults of other regulators, and there are some particular reasons to fear that problems encountered in other regulatory settings will loom larger in a regulated health care system. For one thing, the mystical importance of health care makes it hard for regulators to say "no" to any increment in the quality of care, however small and whatever its hidden cost. And, as I have already noted, the "Roemer effect" supplies a stronger temptation for restricting cost-saving innovation than in other regulated industries, where lesser excuses have nevertheless sufficed to deny consumers the benefits of change.

BENEFITS, COSTS OF ENTRY CONTROLS

With some sense of the probable behavioral characteristics of certification-of-need agencies, it is possible to attempt a final balancing of the benefits and costs of certification-of-need requirements for hospital investments. The conclusion must be that the benefits of such a law seem to have been exaggerated, while potential costs have been largely ignored.

It is a reasonable working hypothesis that certification-of-need agencies will have no incentive to do more than bring about conditions roughly equivalent to those that a hospital cartel would maintain if it could. Cartel-like regulation would foster continued (though somewhat reduced) oversupply rather than the undersupply characteristic of cartels generally, perpetuating excess capacity precisely because of the continuance of the same underlying conditions—third-party cost reimbursement and provider influence over demand—which produce excessive hospital growth in the first place. Indeed, given the strong pressures that act upon certification-of-need agencies, only the best regulatory programs are likely to be effective even to a degree that a provider cartel could approve.

The inescapable conclusion is that, while certification-of-need laws may achieve some reduction in the supply of hospital beds and duplicative services, the public will get substantially less relief than it is entitled to. It is interesting to compare the choice involved in accepting such partial relief with the choices presented by other cartel-like arrangements being offered in solution to the health care industry's problems. For example, PSROs, the so-called foundations for medical care, and other self-regulatory programs may also be analyzed as cartels which, though undeniably dedicated to improving existing conditions somewhat, ultimately will stop well short of delivering to the public all the benefits that a well-organized competitive market (or an appropriately regulated system) would yield. Indeed, it is not inaccurate to view the fundamental health policy choice as being between, on the one hand, a system controlled directly or indirectly by organized providers who accommodate their public responsibilities with their own self-interest and, on the other hand, a system of social control by impersonal market forces, allowing cost-conscious consumers a larger impact and assigning government a less intrusive role. (The difficulty of designing a workable market-oriented solution, while considerable, is no greater than developing an effective regulatory program. However, this is not the place to examine that question.)

Even if one thinks the public should be satisfied with a plan that would control hospital expansion even slightly, there are reasons for doubting that even effective control of supply will have much of a beneficial impact on the cost of health care, which, after all, is the ultimate objective. The argument is simply that, if opportunities exist for raising prices, hospitals may find ways of allowing noncapital expenses, such as personnel costs, to rise even if capital costs and utilization are somehow controlled. Since it is practically impossible to achieve regulatory control of all inputs and their prices, inflationary pressures are apt, like a balloon, to bulge out at another place even if growth in one direction is effectively prevented. In the absence of any affirmative evidence of significant cost-control benefits from certification-of-need laws (and no one has produced any) the possibility that these benefits are no more than minimal must be taken seriously.

Having discounted though perhaps not ruled out hopes for significant benefits from certification of need, we may now look at the opposite side of the cost–benefit ledger. The costs of certification-of-need regulation include (1) significant administrative and compliance costs; (2) losses in efficiency and other benefits (including control of internal subsidization of wasteful, unneeded services) that hospital competition might yield; and (3) as earlier noted, possible serious losses from the retardation of innovation and change (including HMO development and other means of substituting cheaper forms of care for that now being rendered by hospitals). Because by their nature the lost benefits from innovation are impossible to prove convincingly and because regulatory protectionism breeds powerful vested interests, it will be impossible to reverse a legislative decision to regulate entry even if it is in fact a serious mistake. Therefore this loss of policy flexibility is an important added cost of starting down the road to public utility regulation.

While one cannot prove that certification-of-need laws will do more harm than good; they and other regulatory programs directly controlling or restricting entry on principles similar to those underlying public utility regulation must seem unpromising tools for dealing with spiraling health care costs. This is not to say that other kinds of regulation, perhaps including rate regulation, do not have a place in public policies toward health. Nor is it to say that a moratorium on hospital construction might not be wise as part of a temporizing policy designed to curb hospital growth while other, more market-oriented measures take hold. But institutionalized, politically vulnerable mechanisms for excluding new entrants and competitive influences from the health care system seem undesirable at a time when major changes in health care delivery are being sought. Only the narrowest kind of certification-of-need law, adopted as a temporary expedient and not trumpeted as a permanent solution to any problem, can be reconciled with the concerns expressed here. Of much greater long-run importance is attention to developing financing mechanisms that allow and encourage consumers to select their providers on the basis of cost, convenience, and such elements of quality as they can reasonable appraise.

REFERENCES AND NOTES

1. Somers AR: State regulation of hospitals and health care: The New Jersey story, Blue Cross Rep (Res Ser No. 11), July 1973.
2. Havighurst CC: Regulation of health facilities and services by "Certificate of need," Va Law Rev 59:1143, 1973.
3. Green M, Nader R: Economic regulation vs. competition: Uncle Sam the monopoly man, Yale Law J 82:871, 1973.
4. Green M, Nader R: *op. cit.*, p 883.

ALONZO S. YERBY, M.D., M.P.H.
Professor and Head, Department of Health Services Administration
Harvard School of Public Health

Regulation of Health Manpower

Regulation of health manpower has been dominated by the conflict between needs of society for safe and effective medical care and the insistence of the health professionals on autonomy. Of this latter concern, Freidson[1] states:

> The only truly important and uniform criterion for distinguishing professions from other occupations is the fact of autonomy—a position of legitimate control over work. That autonomy is not absolute, depending for its existence upon the toleration and even protection by the state and not necessarily including all zones of activity . . . the single zone of activity in which autonomy *must* exist in order for professional status to exist is in the content of the work itself. . . . In one way or another, through a process of political negotiation and persuasion, society is led to believe that it is desirable to grant an occupation the professional status of self-regulative autonomy.

Professional self-regulation of medicine became institutionalized in the Middle Ages when medical faculties of the universities began to license physicians. Sigerist[2] states that the medical faculty of Salerno licensed physicians early in the thirteenth century. The first medical practice law was also a product of that century when the code of Frederick II, king of Sicily, established educational requirements for physicians and also provided for a sort of internship or a minimal period of postgraduate training.[3]

A milestone in the evolution of governmental recognition of self-regulation of medicine came when a charter was granted to the Royal College of Physicians in England in 1518. In the American colonial period, New Jersey was the first to authorize its medical society to examine candidates for medical practice. Pennsylvania in 1794 considered a bill that would have prescribed educational requirements and required the candidate to present a diploma from a university or college conferring the degree of Doctor or Bachelor of Medicine, or to pass an examination given by a committee composed entirely of physicians. Maryland in 1798 established a Medical Board of Examiners to examine candidates and issue licenses authorizing them to practice medicine.[3]

At present, in the United States, all states have established a state board of medical examiners. In the majority of states the board of medical examiners is appointed by the governor from a list of practicing physicians recommended by the state medical association.[4] All states require a licensing examination, which is separate from and in addition to examinations required for graduating from medical schools. In countries where medical schools are operated or closely supervised by government, successful completion of the required medical curriculum qualifies an individual to practice medicine without a state examination.

Medical licensing boards in the United States are empowered to determine the eligibility of candidates for licensure (including review of character and moral fitness, assessment of educational qualifications, administration of examinations, and approval of postgraduate internships); to accredit or approve medical schools; to issue, register, and renew medical licenses; to decide the recognition to be given to licenses of other jurisdictions; to make administrative rules and regulations concerning professional standards; and to suspend, revoke, and reinstate licenses in disciplinary proceedings.[5]

State boards of medical examiners range in size from 4 to 16 members. In 29 states the boards consist entirely of physicians. In 7 states one or two public members are authorized; however, in 6 of these 7 states the public members are state officials. Sixteen state boards include members of other professions licensed by the board, such as dentists, chiropractors, osteopaths, and veterinarians.

Members of state boards of medical examiners are appointed by the governor or by another official with the governor's approval or confirmation. In 24 states the members are recommended by the state medical society or other professional societies where these professions are licensed by the same board. Only 2 states provide for consultation with or selection by medical educators.

All states require state licensing board members to be licensed practitioners, and most require that a physician member must have practiced in the state for a period of time, usually five years. Eleven states prohibit faculty members or persons connected with educational institutions from serving on medical licensing boards. Several states have repealed the restriction on faculty members serving on boards and one state now requires that one member of the board be a full-time member of the faculty of the University of Illinois College of Medicine.

The review of licensure laws commissioned by the National Advisory Commission on Health Manpower concluded with the following observations:

1. Current statutory provisions impose constraints on medical school curricula innovations;

2. Specific statutory requirements restrain needed developments in graduate medical education, such as elimination of the internship as a separate entity and substitution of appropriate programs of graduate medical education integrated with undergraduate medical education;

3. Initial licensure examination requirements of the states do not measure many of the qualities relevant to fitness to practice and are not necessarily relevant to current goals of undergraduate medical education;

4. Legal requirements for programs in continuing medical education to prevent educational obsolescence are absent;

5. Incomplete interstate recognition of medical licenses results in barriers to geographic mobility of physicians;

6. Licensure requirements for foreign medical graduates are not generally geared specifically to fitness to practice high-quality American medicine;

7. Delegation of tasks to allied and auxiliary personnel is governed by statutes that may be restrictive, ambiguous, or unrelated to accepted custom and usage;

8. Statutory interpretations relevant to delegations of tasks by physicians to allied and auxiliary personnel are not always based on the realities of the delivery of modern medical care;

9. Osteopaths cannot, under present laws, be integrated fully into the practice of medicine so as to permit their addition to the pool of physician manpower; and

10. Attempts to control unscientific schools of practice or cultism by licensure cannot give unscientific practices a scientific basis but

can endanger the public by giving unscientific schools, such as chiropractic, protection through the sanction of law.

The report of the study ends with the observation that the resolution of these problems will require legislative action and, that among the many problems presented by the medical licensure laws, without question the issue of delegation of tasks is a highly significant, if not the most significant, problem requiring resolution.

Since the publication of the Report of the National Advisory Commission on Health Manpower in November of 1967, a number of proposals for reform of the existing practices and legal requirements for licensure of health manpower have been advanced. These include

1. addition or expansion of public members of licensing boards;[6]
2. reorganization of licensing boards;[6]
3. institutional licensure of health personnel;[7–12] and
4. mandatory relicensure.

Public Members of Licensing Boards A number of bills have been introduced in state legislatures to add public members to medical licensing boards. Most of these proposed laws would add one or two public members. Cohen[6] concludes that "the net effects of such token structural change would probably not be far-reaching. . . . It would appear that unless board composition were to be *dramatically* altered, the considerable influence of professional associations on the governance and decision making of licensing boards would continue unchecked by other interests."

Reorganization of Licensing Boards Proposals for reorganizing licensing boards tend to call for consolidation of separate boards into a single board with a subcommittee structure. The subcommittees would have membership majorities from the licensed profession. Other proposals would bring all licensing functions under a single state agency such as a department of health or education. In general, it would appear that these forms of reorganization are unlikely to have any substantial effect on the activities of licensure boards.

Institutional Licensure of Health Personnel Institutional licensure of health personnel is proposed as a substitute for all or a substantial proportion of the licensure of professional and technical manpower. At present health care facilities are licensed or approved by a state agency, usually the state health department. Present licensure requirements deal with such matters as ownership, purpose, organization, and the condition of the physical plant in respect to sanitation, safety, occupancy ratios, and minimal requirements for certain classes of personnel. Institutions providing health care would be given the responsibility of accrediting of personnel.

Proponents of institutional licensure claim that it would help solve the problems created by the rapid proliferation of new groups of health manpower who pressure for licensure as a form of recognition. Concern for this problem is indicated by the action of the American Medical Association and the American Hospital Association in 1970 in adopting resolutions calling for a nationwide moratorium on licensure of additional categories of personnel. The AHA[10] resolution stated:

> Licensing of additional health care occupations will fractionalize further the provision of health services, impede job advancement for employees, and hinder management in utilizing new knowledge and technological advances. The furtherance of health care services depends on a more unified approach for preparing, developing, and using manpower in a safe yet flexible manner.

Hershey[7] calls for the elimination of all individual licensure and the placement of responsibility on institutions for appropriate utilization of personnel in line with educational and experiential qualifications, and in accordance with standards established by potent state institution-licensing agencies. He proposes that the physician's private office and all other facilities that provide health services, such as occupational health facilities, would be subject to regulation as health institutions in regard to the utilization of personnel.

McAdams[8] would have the Joint Commission on Accreditation of Hospitals or a new private agency be responsible for the setting of standards of health personnel rather than Hershey's "potent" state agency.

Lloyd[9] proposed the repeal of all existing laws governing the licensure of health manpower and that there be established new licensure for medicine, dentistry, nursing, medical technology, medical therapy, and institutional licensure. The latter would include administrators, medical record librarians, dietitians, and medical social workers.

The Illinois Hospital Association[13] proposed that present laws be amended to exempt from licensure personnel working in a hospital.

The health insurance proposal of the American Hospital Association[14] would institute a form of institutional licensure in that Health Care Corporations would be established.

> As Ameriplan phases in Health Care Corporations covering geographic areas of each state, the present system of licensure of health personnel should be phased out and the Health Care Corporations made responsible for the competence of all employees.

> The responsibility of the Health Care Corporations for the competency of all their health care personnel would also apply to physicians, dentists, nurses, and pharmacists. Therefore national standards for the measurement of competency of these groups would be indispensable. . . . The Health Care Corporation would rely on this national licensure as a guarantee of basic qualifications.

The Health Security Act proposed by Senator Edward M. Kennedy and Representative Martha Griffiths[15] approaches the concept of institutional licensure of personnel by providing for the establishment of national standards for physicians, dentists, optometrists, podiatrists, and nurses. Physicians, dentists, optometrists, and podiatrists licensed in any state and meeting national standards could practice in any other state. Nurses meeting national standards could practice in any state. A practitioner of any health profession other than medicine or dentistry or any nonprofessional health occupation meeting national standards could work under the supervision of a physician or dentist in any participating public or voluntary hospital or health maintenance organization.

The latter arrangement designed to cover paraprofessional personnel is not unlike Roemer's[16] proposal for the licensure of health teams working in hospitals, extended care facilities, clinics, neighborhood health centers, group practices, laboratories, pharmacies, and other multidisciplinary organizations.

> The head of the team would be licensed as an individual and authorized to supervise certain kinds of unlicensed personnel working in his team, provided certain criteria of good patient care were met. . . . The unlicensed members of the team would be required to meet certain educational qualifications, both initial and continuing.

Presumably the physician would be held responsible for verifying the educational qualifications of the team members and for assuring their participation in continuing education activities.

Tancredi,[11] in an article generally favorable toward the Hershey model of institutional licensure, points out that, because of its sole reliance on input regulation to control the quality of practice, all of the constrictive features of licensure cannot be avoided. He believes that, in spite of its disadvantages, institutional licensure can serve as a bridge to a future stage of regulation characterized by primary reliance on the measurement of treatment outcomes to achieve quality control.

Carlson[12] presents a detailed analysis of licensing and its effect on the quality of care. He concludes by proposing that statutory licensure laws be amended to repeal licensure restrictions for all health care practitioners other than the physician when such practitioners are employed by health care organizations registered to do business in the state and licensed to provide health care. All practitioners not employed by health care organizations should be required to obtain certificates of practice from a health manpower board consisting of representatives of health professions, with a majority of nonprofessional representation. Physician licensure would be retained for all physicians who are not affiliated with health care organizations and even for those physicians who are affiliated with such organizations until such time as geographic mobility would not be impeded by unlicensed status. Physician licensure would then be abolished and replaced by a registry scheme administered by a state health manpower board. Health care organizations would agree to submit to the process and jurisdiction of state courts as a condition of licensure and to participate in a statutory compensation for medical injuries when such a system is developed.

In a thoughtful review of institutional licensure of health personnel Kelley[17] suggests that institutional licensure would create special problems for nurses. She raises questions of supervision, delegation, and the possibility that nurses may be pressured into performing functions for which they are not trained, such as dispensing medication from the pharmacy while on night duty. "Nurses, particularly, who are just beginning to fulfill their potential for total health care, proudly accountable to the patient and not to an administrative hierarchy or a physician for their professional acts, may find themselves relegated to increasing technical tasks, substituting for a more expensive physician."

Addressing the problem of standards and supervision Kelley asks:

> If 50 states cannot now agree on criteria for individual licensure, why would institutional licensure be different? . . . What army of inspectors knowledgeable in all the subcategories of health care can be recruited, employed, and dispersed to check the hundreds of thousands employed in these multiple subcategories [of personnel]—not only in hospitals, but in all other institutions providing health services to the public, such as nursing homes, physicians' offices, clinics. . . ?

Institutional licensure would appear to be a form of decentralization of the state authority over health personnel. However, since state or perhaps national standards would be required, and some means of verifying compliance with such standards would be necessary; responsibility rather than authority would be passed on to health care institutions.

The trend toward the unionization of professional and paraprofessional health workers leads to still another organization (the labor union) with a vested interest in the scope of the work. Institutional licensure could provide employers with an advantage over the labor unions in that the employers' definition of work to be performed would have the support of law and might be deemed not subject to collective bargaining.

It is perhaps significant that most of the proponents of institutional licensure of health personnel are lawyers. Health professional opinion, as evidenced by positions taken by the American Medical Association and the American Nurses Association, appears to be opposed. In considering institutional licensure as a replacement for the present system of professionally dominated licensing boards and certifying societies, health professionals could well bear in mind Freidson's[1] dictum that professional status requires the exercise of autonomy over the content of the work itself.

Finally, institutional licensure would appear to be yet another movement toward bureaucratization of all forms of social interaction. What would be lost if individual responsibility and accountability is subsumed by the institution with the sanction of the state? Is there not a danger that the carrying out of orders would become a substitute for professional judgment, ethics, or the exercise of private conscience?

Mandatory Relicensing of Health Personnel The rapidity with which substantial portions of medical knowledge become obsolete poses a problem for practitioners and regulating bodies. Many health professionals enroll in formal courses offered by the programs of continuing education; others attempt to keep abreast of development by reading scientific journals and attending professional conferences. Some professionals are fortunate enough to work in a setting which ensures maintenance of an adequate knowledge base and technical skills. However, it is generally believed that many (perhaps most) health professionals are unable or unwilling to devote the time and effort to maintain a satisfactory level of competence. This state of affairs has led to proposals for mandatory relicensing.

One state, New Mexico, now requires continuing education as a condition for relicensure of physicians. Dr. Claude Welch,[18] in his inaugural address as president of the American College of Surgeons, predicted mandatory relicensure of physicians within a decade. Dr. Welch stated that recertification could be accomplished through such means as computer re-examinations every five or ten years, individual participation in varied educational activities, or through a peer review system.

The National Advisory Commission on Health Manpower recommended in 1967 that relicensure should be granted either upon a certificate of acceptable performance in continuing education programs or on the basis of challenge examinations in the practitioner's specialty.

Mueller[19] contends it is a physician's performance at work that should be assessed and that periodic examinations like those of Part III of the National Board of Medical Examiners or some of the specialty board examinations are, therefore, inappropriate tools. The goal of a productive life is not continuing education, but continued production. The examination system ought to focus on the results of productive activity and reflect, not the information used, but the processes of patient management and the results of patients managed. This requires a permanent register of procedures and effectiveness drawn from office records, hospital admissions, operative records, tissue reports, medical audits, length of patient's hospital stay, complications, diagnoses, deaths, and other objective areas of physician activity. Every five or ten years there should be a formal reassessment examining the practitioner's information and his use of information. The major component of the reassessment program would be a review of patient results in office, group practice, or hospital records. Mueller contends that peer review has consistently been inadequate to guarantee high standards of physician performance and believes that objective outsiders (lay examiners) acquainted with medical practices, even though unacquainted with specific medical knowledge, would be preferable. It is doubtful that Mueller's proposal will be implemented in the foreseeable future.

The Commission on Professional and Hospital Activities' professional activities study and medical audit programs offer extensive standardized abstracts for all kinds of hospitalized cases, automated information handling and in-depth investigation without access to original records.[20] The National Board of Medical Examiner's programmed testing of patient-management problems[21] and automated problem-centered record systems[22] offer effective tools for objective evaluation of physician performance.

While techniques of evaluation and outcome measurement are being refined and validated, efforts must be directed toward overcoming the resistance of professionals to change in the present system of lifetime licensure.

Licensure of Physicians and the Role of the National Board of Medical Examiners The National Board of Medical Examiners (NBME) is a voluntary organization, established in 1915 with the objective of providing examinations of high quality so that legally established licensing authorities of the states could, at their discretion, license a physician to practice without further examination.[23]

The examinations given by NBME are in three parts: Part I is given to medical students after the completion of the first two (preclinical) years of medical school; Part II is given toward the end of the fourth year of medical school and tests the student's knowledge of clinical medicine; and Part III is given toward the end of the internship and is designed to test clinical competence.

In 1950 NBME abandoned the essay type of examination and adopted objective multiple-choice examinations. With refinement of the examination procedure it became possible to make valid comparisons between the students and graduates of different medical schools. NBME test score averages came to be viewed by many individuals as a useful measure of the quality of medical education. A decline in the standing of Harvard medical students on the 1968 examination contributed to a decision by the faculty of medicine to modify a recently adopted curriculum and to return to the traditional four-level grading system.[24] Forty-eight states and the District of Columbia accept certification by NBME in lieu of the state examination.

Beginning in 1953 with the state of Connecticut, state boards of medical licensure began to use standardized examinations prepared by NBME. Sixteen state boards used NBME examinations in 1967. During that year the Federation of State Medical Boards requested that NBME develop a Federation Licensing Examination (FLEX).[21]

The examination developed for the Federation is scored by NBME, and comparisons are made with performance on NBME examinations. The FLEX examination, like the NBME examination, includes clinical material in the form of color prints of patients, gross and microscopic specimens, roentgenograms, electrocardiograms, charts, and tabular material. The examination also includes programmed testing of the student's ability to manage the clinical problems of patients. Forty-seven states had adopted the FLEX examination by the end of 1973. Hubbard concludes that a logical dual system has evolved, with the NBME examination focused on the student of today who is the physician of tomorrow and the FLEX examination assessing the basic knowledge and clinical competence of the physician of today (the student of earlier years).

A report of a committee on goals and priorities of NBME released in the summer of 1973 recommended that full licensure to practice be deferred until a physician has completed his formal medical education, including specialty training. Upon graduation from medical school the physician would take an examination that would establish his right to provide patient care under supervision. A second examination at the end of specialty training would test his competence in a specific specialty of medicine.

Other recommendations of the Committee include

1. evolution of medical education into a genuine continuum, covering undergraduate, graduate, and post-certification periods; and
2. reorganization of NBME by creating an operational structure composed of five councils: Council for Undergraduate Medical Evaluation, Council for Graduate Medical Evaluation, Council for Evaluation of Continuing Medical Competence, Council for Evaluation of New Health Practitioners, and Council for Research and Development.

The Council for Evaluation of New Health Practitioners would be concerned with assessing the competence of nonphysicians, such as physicians' assistants. The Council for the Evaluation of Continuing Medical Competence would be concerned with the question of periodic relicensure or recertification. NBME is developing examinations for self-assessment programs, which are being offered by specialty societies.[25]

Peer Review and the Regulation of Physicians Professional self-regulation, traditionally a voluntary activity on the part of professional societies, specialty colleges, and the medical staffs of hospitals, has been given the weight of legal authority by the passage by Congress of Public Law 92-603, the Social Security Amendments of 1972. Section 249(F), the Professional Standards Review Organization (PSRO or "Bennett" Amendment–after its sponsor, Senator Wallace Bennett) calls for review of the professional activities of physicians, other health care providers, and institutional providers in the provision of care to beneficiaries under the Social Security Act. Professional Standards Review Organizations will be required to determine whether (1) services provided are medically necessary; (2) the quality of services meets professionally recognized standards of health care; and (3) with respect to the site or level of care, services were provided in the most efficient and effective fashion consistent with the provision of appropriate medical care.[26]

The law requires both retrospective review of services rendered and prospective review of elective admissions to institutions or the provision of costly or lengthy services. A PSRO must maintain and regularly review profiles of services provided by physicians and other health care providers, and of the services received by patients. A PSRO must apply professionally developed norms of care, diagnosis, and treatment, which are based on the patterns of practice in its region. Physicians who are found to be chronic offenders may be denied payment of claims, declared ineligible to participate in the Medicaid or Medicare programs, fined up to $5,000, and have their questionable behavior made public.

While the American Medical Association supports the concept of peer review, individual physicians and some state medical societies have opposed the PSRO program. The House of Delegates of the Indiana State Medical Association adopted a resolution calling for the repeal of the PSRO Amendment to the Social Security Act.

It is difficult to predict what far-reaching effects will flow from this new exercise of governmental authority, which requires that physicians regulate certain of their activities while acting as an agent of the state. Decker and Bonner[27] have concluded:

> PSRO is . . . a managerial tool. It is a governmental plea for medical involvement in the effective and efficient distribution of medical services . . . it is a necessary precursor to the further public assumption of responsibility for the financing of health care. PSRO is organized medicine's opportunity for self-regulation. Given the pressures which now exist for national health insurance, failure of PSRO may well initiate other, less workable forms of bureaucratic control over the practice of medicine.

Other Forms of State Regulation of Health Manpower The regulation of health manpower by the state is not limited to licensure. Public institutions have on occasion imposed requirements in excess of licensure on physician members of their staffs. When these requirements have been challenged in courts of law, some courts have upheld the hospital's action. In *Dade County v. Trombly* (102 So 2d 394–Florida, 1958) the court held that a public hospital had the right to require higher standards for major surgery than the state required license.

In *Green v. City of St. Petersburg* (17 So 2d 517–Florida, 1944) the court held that the plaintiff physician had to conform to the hospital's rules that a surgeon must be on probation for 2 years and thereafter perform 20 major operations under supervision before he could perform major surgery on his own. In an elegant decision the court held the following:

> The practice of major surgery is a highly specialized field and is recognized as a delicate art. The majority of physicians admit that it requires special skill and training and do not (pretend to) enter the field. . . . It is utterly futile to contend in our day that one be permitted to take a scalpel in hand and explore the cranium, the thorax or the abdomen, patch the viscera, remove a tumor or amputate a limb before he demonstrates his qualification to do so. . . .
>
> It would project the doctrine of freedom and equality into unwarranted areas to hold that one could practice major surgery with facilities furnished by the City when he has nothing more than a diploma from a medical school and a certificate from the State Board of Medical Examiners to warrant his skill in that field. A lawyer with these credentials would not be employed to make out a complicated income tax return; a teacher with the equivalent of this would not be employed to

teach Calculus or Theology, . . . and so we might add cases ad infinitum when special training is prerequisite to employment in specialized fields. . . . Constitutional guarantees were not designed to intercept or stalemate progress in these factors; neither were they intended to hamper a community in raising the standard of its schools, hospitals, and other institutions as high as reason and circumstances dictate.

In 1964 the Hospital Code of the City of New York was revised to limit the practice of surgery in proprietary hospitals to qualified surgeons.* In a suit (*Ferrante v. City of New York*, 1964) the New York Supreme Court cited studies made prior to 1964 that revealed serious deficiencies in the quality of the medical and surgical services performed in proprietary hospitals and dismissed as being without merit the contention by the plaintiff (Dr. Ferrante) that the imposition of qualifications for performing surgery at proprietary hospitals that he could not meet was unconstitutional.

Dr. Ferrante, merely by virtue of his license to practice medicine in New York State and his having performed surgery for many years in proprietary hospitals, did not acquire a vested constitutional right to continue to perform surgery in such hospitals. Whatever rights he possessed were subject and subordinate to the right of the appropriate public authorities to require that physicians performing surgery in hospitals possess requirements calculated to protect the public from the dangers of surgery at the hand of incompetent and unqualified practitioners.

These decisions rather than representing intrusion of the courts into the practice of medicine, are reaffirmations of society's compact with the health care system that it must exercise the ultimate responsibility for standards of competence.

Regulation of Allied Health Manpower The term *allied health manpower* is used to cover all professional, technical, and supportive workers in the fields of patient care, community health, public health, environmental health, and related health research, who engage in activities that support, complement, or supplement the professional functions of administrators and practitioners.[28]

Estimates of the number of professional, technical, or vocational specialties that can be identified as components of allied health manpower vary from 100[28] to over 200.[29] The rapid proliferation of new occupational groups has resulted in the employment of a variety of

*In New York a *qualified surgeon* is a physician holding a current license to practice medicine in the State of New York and who is a Diplomate of the American Board of Surgery, a Fellow of the American College of Surgeons, eligible for examination by the American Board of Surgery, or has completed an approved residency in surgery or holds the rank of attending or Associate Attending Surgeon in an accredited voluntary or governmental hospital.

legal and voluntary means of regulating or certifying them. These include state licensure, certification by a professional or technical society, or recognition of the graduates of accredited programs.

A number of writers oppose licensing of allied manpower. They point out that most licenses are issued upon examination after completion of professional or occupational training, and as yet little progress has been made toward mandatory relicensure-based assurance of continued competence.[30] Others have expressed concern that states have initiated licensing activity for a class of personnel before any students have been accepted in an educational or training program and before the occupation seeks it.[31]

Curran[32] examined the Colorado "Child Health Associate Law." The act requires that a pediatrician must be approved to supervise an associate and may supervise only one at a time. The associate must practice as an employee of the pediatrician within the physical quarters of his professional office and only when the pediatrician is "directly and personally available." The associate may practice outside the professional office if in the "direct and personal presence" of the employing pediatrician, or in "follow-up care of a patient pursuant to the specific directions of such physician related to that particular patient." Such associates may be employed by public, governmental agencies, but not by private or voluntary agencies or hospitals. This scope of activity seems more restrictive than would normally be true of a well-trained public health nurse doing bedside care in a community. A high price for granting licensure to this new group has been extracted by this legislation. Curran points out that this strict control is in the form of a license law and not a registration act and as such it outlaws all use of such pediatric assistants except under the provisions of the act.

> No other experimental programs to produce similar personnel can be developed in Colorado, or be imported from other states, except in accordance with these detailed precepts. A registration act, on the other hand, could have been adopted which would have provided the same recognition to this particular group of trainees, the same legal protection to the group, but without outlawing similar experiments that do not carry the same title or credentials. . . . In general, it is best in the evolution of professional groups to begin with registration acts and move to full, mandatory licensure only after the professional group is fully matured, clearly defined in its own responsibilities, and capable within its own educational and training programs of meeting the reasonable manpower needs in its field of practice.

Curran cites the California "Physician's Assist" law as being a considerable improvement of the Colorado Child Health Associate Law. The California law is a registration act that allows the State Board of

Medical Examiners to approve the employment of physician's assistants who have completed approved training programs. The board may develop criteria and standards for such programs. The law specifically allows and *encourages* the utilization of equivalencies and proficiency testing to give full credit to trainees for previous education and experience. The law simply authorizes "medical services" to be performed under the supervision of a physician or physicians approved by the board. A physician may supervise no more than two assistants. Curran concludes that this law is the best that he has seen in the field and recommends it as a model for other states considering such legislative measures.

Dye[33] opposes separate independent licensure of physician assistants on the grounds that the resulting new type of licensed practitioner would bring about a marked diminution of the control of the practice of medicine by state medical boards. Donelson[34] advocated licensure of physicians' assistants to work under the direct supervision and control of physicians. Egelston and Kinser[29] maintain that neither strict enforcement of existing laws or continued licensure of existing and emerging occupations seems to be in the best interest of patients, employers, or employees. They point out that professional groups and employers resist the use of certification. Professional groups charge that there is no way to enforce an employer's acceptance of a certified graduate of a training program, and that hospital authorities argue that educational requirements established by educators or professional groups do not necessarily match job performance requirements.

Certification Certification is a form of voluntary regulation of health manpower. Certification is carried out by professional associations on the basis of prescribed qualification of education or experience. Some professional associations also require and administer a qualifying examination.

Certification has been the major form of regulation of allied health manpower. The U.S. Department of Health, Education, and Welfare report on Accreditation and Certification[35] lists 28 nongovernmental academies, associations, boards, and registries that certify allied health personnel. Some of the professional associations were organized in the early decades of this century. The International Association of Milk, Food, and Environmental Sanitarians was founded in 1911, and the American Dietetic Association and the American Occupational Therapy Association were founded in 1917.

Certification permits a certain degree of flexibility such as the practice of registering, for a limited period of time, experienced people who may not meet the educational requirements. Some certifying groups

(American Dietetic Association) require continuing education to maintain registration.

Specialty certification in medicine, dentistry, osteopathy, and veterinary medicine is carried out by specialty boards recognized by the respective national professional associations. These boards uniformly require that diplomates have graduate education, a period of supervised experience, recognized competency, and the successful completion of an examination given by the board. One specialty board, the American Board of Internal Medicine, has announced that it will award a qualifying certificate to candidates who pass the examination, but candidates will be subject to a requirement of renewal.[36] The board is moving toward a definite recertification procedure and its progress is likely to be closely followed by other specialty boards.

CONCLUDING OBSERVATIONS

Societies have sought to ensure the safety and effectiveness and moral rectitude of the healing professions since the emergence of these specialized classes of healers. Execution, maiming, or blinding the faltering practitioner have long since given way to prescribed education and training with some form of official license or credential as evidence of compliance. The quality and quantity of specialized knowledge required by healers forced societies to relinquish control to the practitioners. The granting of control to the professionals is a fiduciary commitment and, if violated, the mandate may be withdrawn. At this point in history in this society the message appears to be—control will increasingly be shared.

REFERENCES AND NOTES

1. Freidson E: Profession of Medicine. New York, Dodd, Mead, and Company, 1970. 407 pp.
2. Sigerist HE: The history of medical licensure. J Am Med Assoc 104:1056–1060, 1935, reprinted in Roemer MI, ed: Henry Sigerist on the Sociology of Medicine. New York, M.D. Publications, 1960. 397 pp.
3. Derbyshire RC: Medical Licensure and Discipline in the United States. Baltimore, The Johns Hopkins Press, 1969. 183 pp.
4. Roemer R: Legal systems regulating health personnel, Milbank Mem Fund Q, 46:431–471, 1968.
5. Forgotson E, Roemer R, Newman RW: Legal regulation of health personnel in the United States. Appendix VII of Report of the National Advisory Commission on Health Manpower, Vol. II. Washington, D.C., U.S. Government Printing Office, 1967.

6. Cohen HS: Professional licensure, organizational behavior and the public interest. Health Soc 51:73–88, 1973.
7. Hershey N: The inhibiting effect upon innovation of the prevailing licensure system. Ann NY Acad Sci 166:951–956, 1969.
8. McAdams D: Institution-based licensure system may help solve the licensure dilemma. Hosp Prog 50:52, 1969.
9. Lloyd JJ: Arguments for state regulation of health professions. Hosp Prog 51:71, 1970.
10. American Hospital Association: Statement on licensure of health care personnel. Hospitals 45:82, 1971.
11. Tancredi LR: The social control of medical practice: Licensure versus output monitoring. Milbank Mem Fund Q 50:99–125, 1972. Part 1.
12. Carlson RH: Health manpower licensing and emerging institutional responsibility for quality of care. Law Contemp Probl 35:849–878, 1970.
13. Illinois Hospital Association: Hospitals, manpower, licensure and the 1970's. Chicago, Illinois Hospital Association, 1971 (mimeographed).
14. Ameriplan—A Proposal for the Delivery and Financing of Health Services in the United States. Report of a Special Committee on the Provision of Health Services. Chicago, American Hospital Association, 1970.
15. The Health Security Program, S.3., 93rd Congress.
16. Roemer R: Licensing and regulation of medical and medical-related practitioners in health service teams. Med Care 9:42–54, 1971.
17. Kelley, LY: Institutional licensure. Nurs Outlook 21:566–572, 1973.
18. ACS head foresees MD relicensure (Dr. Claude Welch). AMA News, October 29, 1973.
19. Mueller CB: Continuing assessment of medical performance: Proposals for a recertification examination structure. N Engl J Med 284:1378–1380, 1971.
20. Slee V: Information systems and measurement tools. J Am Med Assoc 196 (12):1063–1065, 1966.
21. Hubbard JP: Measuring Medical Education. Philadelphia, Lea & Febiger, 1971. 180 pp.
22. Weed LL: Medical Records, Medical Education and Patient Care. Cleveland, Case Western Reserve University Press, 1971.
23. Womack NA: The evolution of the National Board of Medical Examiners. J Am Med Assoc 192:817, 1965.
24. Goldhaber SZ: Medical education: Harvard reverts to tradition. Science 181: 1027–1032, 1973.
25. Walsh J: Medical evaluation: Design for a comprehensive system. Science 181:1023–1026, 1973.
26. Kavet J, Luft HS: The Implications of the PSRO Legislation for the Teaching Hospital Sector. Boston, Harvard University, Center for Community Health and Medical Care, 1973. 37 pp. (Health Care Policy Discussion Paper, Ser No. B)
27. Decker B, Bonner P: PSRO: Organization for Regional Peer Review. Cambridge, Ballinger Publishing Company, 1973, p. 7.
28. USDHEW NIH Division of Allied Health Manpower: The Allied Health Professions Personnel Training Act of 1966 as Amended; Report to the President and the Congress. Bethesda, Md., National Institutes of Health, 1969. 94 pp.

29. Egelston JF, Kinser T: Licensure of hospital personnel (Part 1). Hospitals 44:35–39, 1970. Licensure and career mobility (Part 2). Hospitals 44:42–46, 1970.
30. Ballenger MD: Physician's assistants and the licensing issue. Mon Labor Rev 94:62–63, 1973.
31. Coleman FC: Licensure problems of allied health personnel. Fed Bull 57:204–213, 1970.
32. Curran W: Health services manpower roadblocks: Legislative measures to facilitate the development of allied manpower roles. Paper delivered at APHA Annual Meeting, Houston, Texas, October 26, 1970. 20 pp (mimeographed).
33. Dye P: State medical boards and statutory provisions in the utilization of professional assistants. Fed Bull 58:274–482, 1971.
34. Donelson MJ: Official status for physician's assistants. Va Med Mon 96.
35. Pennell M, Proffitt J, Hatch T: Accreditation and Certification in Relation to Allied Health Manpower. Bethesda, Md, Bureau of Health Manpower Education, 1971. 43 pp. (NIH Publ No. 71-192)
36. Hickman JB: Periodic recertification. J Am Med Assoc 213:1657–1658, 1970.

IV

Regulation of Payment to Institutions

Two decades of rapidly rising costs for hospital care have attracted the professional attention of economists and regulatory agencies, among many others. Ralph Berry, an economist, explains in this section why he concludes that the increases result largely from increasing demand. As a corollary, he suggests how cost containment can best deal with the factor of demand, in view of that factor's effect on behavior of the hospital industry, which is to inspire more costly services. Harold Cohen describes the experiences of the Maryland Health Services Cost Review Commission in setting up procedures for regulation of hospital and other provider institution rates. The questions raised in the process are widely applicable to any effort for control of charges by health institutions.

Panelists who discussed these two papers were Stuart Altman, Ph.D., deputy assistant secretary for planning and evaluation, Department of Health, Education, and Welfare; Olga Boikess, J.D., of Galland, Kharasch, Calkins, and Brown, attorneys, Washington, D.C.; and David Hitt, chief operating officer, Baylor University Medical Center, Houston.

RALPH E. BERRY, JR., Ph.D.
Associate Professor of Economics, Harvard School of Public Health

Perspectives on Rate Regulation

The cost of hospital care has been rising rapidly for more than 20 years. The average cost per patient day in nonfederal short-term general hospitals, for example, is approximately 6 times as high as it was 20 years ago. Further, the rate of increase of hospital cost has generally been accelerating. The average cost per patient day doubled during the decade of the 1950s. During the decade of the 1960s, the rate of increase was such that cost doubled in 8½ years. The most recent doubling of costs occurred over a span of only 5 years. Hospital cost inflation is not a recent problem, but represents a phenomenon with a rather long history that has displayed a marked tendency to intensify in recent years.

As hospital costs have risen, and particularly as these costs have been translated into a burden through the government budget, more and more pressure has been brought to bear to control these costs. A variety of proposals designed to effect a control on hospital costs has appeared or reappeared in recent years. Incentive reimbursement mechanisms, prospective budgeting, areawide planning, certification of need, and even structural reform of the medical care sector have been suggested as reasonable solutions to the cost problem. Rate regulation is an alternative mechanism for cost control and has been in effect on a national scale under the Economic Stabilization Program for the past 2½ years.

What are the prospects under rate regulation in the hospital industry?

The answer to that question derives from the answers to several more fundamental questions. What is the structure of the hospital industry? What behavioral patterns are associated with varying market conditions? What are the dimensions of the problem of hospital cost inflation? What impact will rate regulation have on structure, behavior, costs, and productivity? The purpose of this paper is to outline certain reflections on these issues and to consider rate regulation in the hospital industry from an economic perspective.

LONG-TERM PRICE TRENDS

Inflation is not unique to the hospital sector; the American economy has been characterized by varying degrees of inflation for more than two decades. In fact, the relative inflation of hospital costs can be put into perspective by comparing it with the general inflation in consumer prices. The data in Table 1 reflect the trends in consumer prices in general and the cost of hospital care specifically over the period 1950–1970.

These data suggest three considerations. First, the choice of price and cost indexes for hospitals implicitly assumes that short-term general and other special hospitals should be the focus of concern for inflation in the hospital sector. Second, it is clear from these data that inflation in the hospital sector seems to vary with general inflation. Third, although the rates of inflation tend to move in the same direction, inflation in the hospital sector has exceeded general inflation by a significant order of magnitude.

It seems appropriate to concentrate on short-term general hospitals in the context of inflation, given the structure of the hospital sector and secular trends in demand. Within the hospital sector there are four

TABLE 1 Average Annual Percentage Increases in Consumer Prices and Hospital Costs

	Percent Increase			
	1950–1955	1955–1960	1960–1965	1965–1970
Consumer Price Index	2.2	2.0	1.3	4.2
Hospital daily service charge	6.9	6.3	5.8	13.9
Average cost per patient day[a]	8.2	6.9	6.7	12.7
Average cost per admission[a]	7.2	6.4	8.9	12.3

SOURCE: Consumer Price Index and hospital daily service charge, *in* Consumer Price Index. Washington, D.C., Bureau of Labor Statistics; Average cost data, *in* Hospital Statistics 1972. Chicago, American Hospital Association.

[a]In nonfederal short-term general and other special hospitals.

distinct subsectors or industries: (1) all short-term general and other special hospitals; (2) all long-term general and other special hospitals; (3) all psychiatric hospitals; and (4) all tuberculosis hospitals. The data in Table 2 reflect the relative dominance of short-term general hospitals.

By any measure, the short-term general hospitals dominate. They represent 87.5 percent of all hospitals, 97 percent of all admissions, more than 60 percent of all beds and the aggregate average daily census, and most significant, perhaps, almost 85 percent of the total expenditures on hospital care in the United States. The focus of concern on short-term general hospitals in the context of cost containment does certainly seem warranted by the relative orders of magnitude involved. Further, the relative dominance of the short-term general hospitals within the sector has increased consistently in recent years.

The most marked increases in demand have occurred in the markets for services provided by short-term general and other special hospitals. Whether utilization is measured by total admissions or by the average daily census, the short-term general hospital industry experienced significant pressure from increased demand during the decade of the 1960s. From 1960 to 1970, total admissions to short-term general hospitals increased by 27.3 percent, and the average daily census increased by 38.8 percent.

The supply of short-term general hospital services has increased, but probably not as much as has demand for them. The number of hospitals increased by 8.4 percent from 1960 to 1970. More significant, the number of beds in short-term general hospitals increased by 32.7 percent. An increase in the overall occupancy rate from 74.7 percent to 78 percent may have compensated partially for the difference between the rates of increase of the average daily census and the number of beds, but the average length of stay was somewhat higher in 1970 (8.2 days) than it had been in 1960 (7.6 days).

Although these changes reflect a variety of factors, such as the scope and quality of care, patterns of practice, and changing patient mix, they serve to indicate the pressure on short-term hospital facilities from increased demand over the long run.

In contrast to the marked upward shift in utilization of short-term general hospitals, the utilization of long-term general and other special hospitals and tuberculosis hospitals has undergone secular decline. Admissions to psychiatric hospitals actually increased by a greater percentage than those to short-term general hospitals, but changing technology, particularly drug and shock therapy, made it possible for psychiatric hospitals to treat an increased number of patients with a significant reduction in the quantity of facilities by drastically lower-

TABLE 2 Facilities and Utilization in the Hospital Sector in 1972

	Hospitals		Beds		Admissions		Average Daily Census		Total Expenses	
Hospital Type	No.	Percent	No. (1000)	Percent	No. (1000)	Percent	No. (1000)	Percent	Amount ($100,000)	Percent
Short-term general and other special	6180	87.5	967	62.3	32,287	97.0	728	60.2	27,728	84.9
Long-term general and other special	249	3.5	80	5.2	287	0.9	67	5.5	1,248	3.8
Psychiatric	559	7.9	490	31.6	659	2.0	407	33.6	3,547	10.9
Tuberculosis	73	1.1	14	0.9	33	0.1	8	0.7	144	0.4
TOTAL	7061	100.0	1551	100.0	33,266	100.0	1210	100.0	32,677	100.0

SOURCE: Hospital Statistics 1972. Chicago, American Hospital Association.

ing the average length of stay. The average daily census of psychiatric hospitals declined by some 33.5 percent from 1960 to 1970.

Not only do short-term general hospitals dominate the hospital sector, but there have also been marked differences in the secular trends in demand for the several types of hospital care. The increase in pressure is unique to the facilities providing essentially short-term services. On balance, increased demand has undoubtedly contributed in part to the inflationary trend in prices for short-term general hospital services.

As noted before, the data in Table 1 indicate that hospital inflation has varied with general inflation over a rather extended period. When the average annual percentage increase in consumer prices declined in the second half of the 1950s and again in the first half of the 1960s, the rate of increase in hospital prices and costs tended to decline as well. When the rate of increase of consumer prices went up significantly during the last half of the 1960s, the rate of increase of hospital prices and cost displayed an equally dramatic increase.

Can hospital cost inflation be attributed largely to the general inflation in the economy? If it could, the issue of cost containment for the hospital sector would have many fewer dimensions. Incentive reimbursement, prospective budgeting, rate regulation, and the like would be relatively cosmetic as regards cost control. There would be no special problem of hospital cost inflation. But few would specifically ascribe the inflation in hospital prices and costs to the general price inflation. Because inflation in the hospital sector has exceeded general inflation for an extended period by a significant order of magnitude, an alternative explanation is needed.

One such alternative, which is a variation on the theme that general inflation causes hospital inflation, is that hospital inflation has occurred as a consequence of the inflation in the costs of inputs that hospitals employ. This explanation has an apparent intuitive appeal to many. Labor costs are particularly significant to hospitals and, it has been argued, not only have hospital wages increased over time to keep pace with the general inflation, but hospital wages have also had to increase more rapidly than wages in general because they were below average for such a long period. The relative rise in hospital wages has often been described as a process of "catching up" with wage levels in the rest of the economy. There are those who have held that the inflation in the hospital sector is a cost-push inflation.

If cost-push inflation is in fact the problem, then the cost containment problem should be viewed in such a context. In the extreme, wage controls would be in order and price controls on inputs employed by hospitals would alleviate hospital inflation, but limitations on the prices of hospital outputs would not control inflation and could serve to exacerbate the problem if wage and price controls on hospital inputs were less than completely effective.

The prices that hospitals must pay for their inputs clearly have risen over time, but does this represent a cause of inflation or a consequence of inflation?

The data in Table 3 reflect the trends in payroll costs, wages, and personnel employed per patient day over the period 1950–1970. These data are not completely consistent with a cost-push hypothesis of hospital inflation. Although the rates of increase of payroll costs and wages have tended to vary with general inflation over the period, two factors are not explained by reference to input cost increases as the fundamental cause of inflation. First, the rates of increase appear to be significantly higher than the general inflation rates in each period. Second, only part of the increase in labor costs was due to higher wages; there has been a significant increase in the number of hospital employees.

One might be tempted to think of the higher rates of increase of wages and labor costs as representing the impact of the "catching-up" process, but that would leave the increase in the quantity of labor employed per patient day unexplained. Further, if the trend in the rate of increase of wages through 1965 represented a closing of the gap between hospital wages and the wages in the rest of the economy, why did the rate of increase accelerate so rapidly in the period 1965–1970?

These questions are interesting in their own right, but they take on added significance in the context of rate regulation and cost containment policy in general. If wage inflation was the primary cause of hospital inflation, exacerbated by the catching-up process, we might expect hospital inflation to be moderated greatly when hospital wages approximated other wages for similar occupations in the economy. But, as the gap between hospital wages and other wages closed, there was no moderation in the rate of hospital inflation; instead the rate of inflation in the hospital sector increased.

TABLE 3 Average Annual Percentage Increases in Payroll Costs, Wages, and Personnel in Nonfederal, Short-Term General Hospitals

	Average Annual Increase (%)			
	1950–1955	1955–1960	1960–1965	1965–1970
Payroll costs per patient day	10.0	7.1	6.5	11.5
Average annual wage rate	7.1	4.8	4.7	7.8
Personnel per patient day	2.7	2.2	1.7	3.4

SOURCE: Hospital Statistics 1972. Chicago, American Hospital Association.

The view among many economists for some time has been that inflation in the hospital sector was primarily caused by increasing demand, that the inflation in hospital costs could be characterized as demand-pull inflation. It was held that higher real incomes, population growth, a change in population mix, and most especially an increase in both private and public insurance coverage have led to an increase in the demand for hospital care. The increase in demand has led to higher prices; higher prices have led to an increase in net revenues earned by hospitals; and these higher revenues have been employed in large part to increase the quality and complexity of the scope of services provided with a consequent increase in the cost of hospital care over time.

Recent empirical studies[1] have essentially confirmed that hospital inflation is indeed a demand-pull inflation. On balance, cost containment policy is more likely to alleviate or moderate hospital cost inflation if mechanisms are developed to come to grips specifically with the impact of demand on the short-term general hospital industry and more especially with the behavioral patterns within the industry.

SOME EVIDENCE FROM TRENDS IN THE 1960s

The introduction of the Medicare program in 1966 was designed to remove the financial barrier to medical care for the nation's elderly citizens. Subject to certain limitations, the program was financially responsible for the hospital expenses of almost 20 million people over the age of 65. In the vernacular of the economist, the price and income constraints were removed for a significant proportion of all consumers. Thus, the immediate impact of the Medicare program on the hospital sector was an increase in demand. What effect did that increase in demand have on hospital behavior, and on prices, costs, net revenues, and productivity?

Profit-motivated hospitals might be expected to react to an increase in demand in much the same way as profit-motivated firms in any other industry. But profit-motivated hospitals constitute an exceedingly small proportion of the hospital sector. At the time of the introduction of the Medicare program, for-profit hospitals provided only 5.6 percent of all short-term general inpatient days. The impact of the Medicare program has to be understood rather in terms of the reaction of nonprofit hospitals to an increase in demand.

A number of economists[2] have concerned themselves in recent years with behavioral models of nonprofit hospitals. It is not the purpose at present to develop a formal model to describe the market behavior of a nonprofit hospital. Rather it should suffice to describe the common interest of those who contribute to the decision-making process of hospitals in the prestige of the institution.

Decision making is the province, to greater or lesser degree, of three groups within a representative hospital—the board of trustees, the medical staff, and the administrator. Each of these is primarily concerned with the prestige of the institution in terms of size, quality, and scope of services. Given a choice, the members of the board of trustees, the members of the medical staff, and the administrator would all prefer a larger hospital, a higher quality hospital, and a hospital providing a more complex scope of services. Of course there are trade-offs among these three objectives, but it is not necessary to specify the trade-offs for present purposes.

As profit-motivated hospitals will react to an increase in demand in a way that would increase their profits, nonprofit hospitals will react to an increase in demand in a way that will increase their prestige.

If these behavioral assumptions are accurate, then an increase in demand for hospital services should lead to an increase in hospital size, the addition of quality-enhancing facilities and services, and an increase in the complexity of the scope of services that individual hospitals provide.

It may be instructive to consider a simple example. Assume that at a point in time there is equilibrium in the market for hospital services and all hospital beds are full. Assume an increase in demand such that with the same number of beds equilibrium requires an increase in price. Now if all hospitals were profit-motivated, profits would rise in the short run and in the long run the supply of hospital services would increase because of their profitability. The reaction of the profit-motivated hospitals to the demand stimulus would be to offer more of the same services. But if all (or some) of the hospitals were prestige-motivated, surplus (profit) would rise in the short run and, in the long run, the supply of hospital services would increase not only in quantity but also in quality and complexity. In fact, for a given surplus (profit), the greater the increase in quality and complexity, the less will be the increase in the quantity of hospital services.

The increase in demand implicit in the introduction of the Medicare program did lead to an increase in the quantity of hospital services supplied, but it led also to increases in the quality of services and increases in the complexity of services provided. The quantity response in the supply of hospital services is implicit in the increases in the number of nonfederal short-term general hospitals, the number of beds, and the average hospital size from 1965 to 1970 as summarized in Table 4.

TABLE 4 Nonfederal Short-Term General Hospitals, Beds, and Average Size, 1965 and 1970

Year	No. Hospitals	No. Beds	Average Bed Size
1965	5736	741,000	129
1970	5859	848,000	145

SOURCE: Hospital Statistics 1972. Chicago, American Hospital Association.

The increases in the quality and complexity of services provided cannot be documented as directly but are implicit in the data summarized in Table 5, which indicate the percentage of hospitals reporting the availability of representative facilities and services that can be characterized as quality-enhancing services and complexity-expanding services.

This phenomenon of nonprofit behavior can lead to an inflationary spiral in the price of hospital services. Consider the obvious extension of the above example in the context of the Medicare program. The increase in demand arises from the removal of price and income constraints for the aged. The increase in demand leads to an increase in prices and surpluses in the short run. The demand is for more hospital places, but the supply response is only in part more hospital places; a significant part of the supply response takes the form of higher quality and more complexity. There will be excess demand until the quantity of hospital services expands to satisfy the Medicare demand. Since the

TABLE 5 Percent of Hospitals Reporting the Availability of Representative Facilities and Services in 1965 and 1970

	Percent Hospitals	
Facilities and Services	1965	1970
Quality-enhancing services		
Blood bank	61.4	60.4
Pharmacy with pharmacist	58.5	83.1
Postoperative recovery room	69.0	75.2
Complexity-expanding services		
Electroencephalography	27.7	33.0
Physical therapy	51.7	61.9
Intensive care unit	26.7	48.8
Radioisotope	30.1	36.1
Cobalt therapy	10.5	12.6

SOURCE: Hospitals (Guide Issue, Part Two), August 1, 1966 and 1971.

program serves to remove the price constraint, this demand will persist, prices will rise, surpluses will rise, and further increases in quality and complexity will occur. (The spiral will be damped to the extent that those consumers for whom the price constraint is not removed are "bid out of the market.")

To the extent that the Medicare program and other third-party sources of hospital revenues reimburse hospitals for "reasonable costs," the new equilibrium will be one characterized by a higher price and cost since the new product will be characterized by higher quality and more complexity. Given the hypothesized behavior of nonprofit hospitals, the extent to which increased demand in general and the Medicare program in particular contributed to inflation can be inferred from the data in Tables 6 and 7. On balance, the pattern is consonant with the structure and behavior outlined above.

TABLE 6 Average Annual Percentage Increases in Prices, Costs, and Real Inputs in Nonfederal Short-Term General Hospitals, 1960–1970

	Average Annual Increase (%)	
	1960–1965	1965–1970
Hospital daily service charge	5.8	13.9
Average cost per patient day	6.7	12.7
Average cost per admission	8.9	12.3
Personnel per patient day	1.7	3.4
Nonlabor inputs per patient day[a]	6.6	11.6
Real inputs per patient day[b]	3.7	6.5

SOURCE: Hospital daily service charge, *in* Consumer Price Index. Washington, D.C., Bureau of Labor Statistics; Average cost data and personnel data, *in* Hospital Statistics 1972. Chicago, American Hospital Association.

[a]Calculated by deflating nonlabor costs per patient day by the Wholesale Price Index.

[b]Calculated by deflating labor costs per patient day by an index of average hospital wages and nonlabor costs per patient day by the Wholesale Price Index and forming a weighted average with 1960 labor and nonlabor ratios of total expenses as weights.

TABLE 7 Average Annual Net Revenues in Nonfederal Short-Term General Hospitals, 1960–1970

	1960–1965	1966–1970
Net revenue: total revenue	2.0	3.2
Net revenue: plant assets	1.5	2.9

SOURCE: Hospitals (Guide Issue, Part Two), August 1, 1961 through 1971.

The rates of increase of prices, costs, and inputs were consistently higher in the second half of the decade than they were in the first half. Similarly, the average annual net revenues, whether measured as a proportion of total revenues or of plant assets, were substantially higher in the years 1966 through 1970 than they were in the years 1960 through 1965.

The increased demand for hospital care, stimulated in large part by the introduction of the Medicare program, had the predicted consequences. Hospital prices, represented by the daily service charge, increased rather dramatically. Average costs increased significantly, but not quite as rapidly as prices. The difference in the rates of increase of prices and costs led to a significant increase in the net revenues of hospitals. Finally, undoubtedly financed in part by the higher net revenues, hospitals increased the quantities of both labor and nonlabor inputs per patient day.*

These, then, are the dimensions of the problem of hospital cost inflation. The various proposals for cost containment should be assessed in terms of the structure of the hospital industry and the behavioral patterns associated with varying market conditions.

INCENTIVE REIMBURSEMENT: DEVELOPMENTS AND PROSPECTS

As hospital costs have risen, and as these costs have been translated into a burden through the budgets of private and public third-party payers, more and more pressure has been brought to bear to control those costs. A variety of proposals designed to effect a control on hospital costs have been put forward. Incentive reimbursement mechanisms, prospective budgeting, areawide planning, certification of need, rate regulation, and structural reform of the medical sector have been proposed to cope with the cost problem. Each of these approaches has some merit; none is likely to be a panacea. Since all of these approaches have been discussed and debated in detail elsewhere, the present purpose is not to attempt a detailed description or analysis of any particular plan or even type of plan, but rather to reflect briefly, in somewhat general terms, on the development and prospects in the context of incentive reimbursement and rate regulation.

*At this point, no judgment is intended as to whether these increases were appropriate or inappropriate, desirable or undesirable, only that they occurred. It should be obvious, for example, that to the extent that the Medicare patients represented a different patient mix with different medical requirements, some part of the increase in inputs can be ascribed to a change in the character of the product produced by hospitals. We will return to this issue later.

Incentive reimbursement as an alternative for cost control in the hospital sector came into national focus when the Social Security Act was amended in 1967 to stimulate such programs. Actually, only a small number of proposals for incentive-reimbursement experiments have been funded by the Social Security Administration, and to date, no program-wide incentive-reimbursement mechanism has evolved or been seriously considered for adoption. Many Blue Cross plans have conducted incentive-reimbursement experiments and several have built incentive reimbursements into their contracts with member hospitals. Still others have been involved in the general development of incentive-reimbursement mechanisms, including certain prepaid group practices, medical foundations, and a limited number of state rate-setting commissions.

The term *incentive reimbursement* represents a rather broad spectrum of activities that are tied directly or indirectly to reimbursement. The essence of the incentive-reimbursement approach is to provide incentives, usually to individual providers, to hold costs down. Conceptually, either positive or negative inducements can be applied, and any factor that affects cost or cost inflation is a potential candidate for incentive reimbursement. Efforts have been directed to affect the demand for care, the expansion of facilities and services, and the relative efficiency of providing care.

Under one experiment funded by the Social Security Administration, a cadre of nurses has been trained to help Medicare patients secure the appropriate amount of care. This represents an attempt to provide an incentive to control demand by avoiding inappropriate demand. In the same general category of controlling demand through incentives, several Blue Cross plans have employed incentives to induce member hospitals to reduce lengths of stay, develop outpatient alternatives, and a variety of similar utilization review activities.

Given the role that increased demand has had in stimulating hospital cost inflation, it is appropriate to direct attention to the demand for hospital care. Certainly unnecessary utilization should be avoided, and efforts such as these should probably be extended. To date, no definitive evaluation of these experiments is available, but it is unlikely that incentive reimbursement is the policy tool with the maximum potential for controlling hospital inflation by controlling demand, even inappropriate demand. On balance, it would appear that, although utilization review is a most appropriate policy and is undoubtedly enhanced by incentive reimbursement, controlling inflation by controlling demand will require certain structural reforms in the medical care sector.

Areawide planning and certification of need have evolved essentially to cope with the expansion of facilities, programs, and equipment beyond those characteristically needed by some definition. In effect, given the behavioral assumptions outlined in the previous section, hospital cost inflation is directly related to the expansion of facilities, programs, and equipment. In many instances, incentive reimbursement has been integrated with areawide planning and certification of need. Several Blue Cross plans require prior approval from areawide planning agencies for the addition of new facilities and services. Usually the incentives involved are negative; that is, reimbursement is refused or reduced when "unnecessary" facilities and services are added. Conceptually, the combination of areawide planning, certification of need, and incentive reimbursement is a potentially powerful policy tool for controlling inflation by controlling the expansion of facilities and services. In practice, the planning agencies and efforts are quite diverse in effectiveness. Again, no definitive evaluation of these experiments is available, but it is clear that the superimposition of incentive reimbursement on planning efforts in general should greatly strengthen the mechanism. Incentive reimbursement *could* represent the missing teeth that have been lamented so often.

Several incentive-reimbursement approaches have evolved that might best be characterized as promoting institutional efficiency. In certain cases, the center of focus has been on individual departments and the general principle is to provide an incentive to employ specific industrial engineering techniques to improve the relative efficiency of the production process and hence effect the desired impact on costs. A somewhat related development involves incentive payments to individual hospitals that compare favorably in terms of cost increases with weighted average cost increases of similar hospitals. In effect, hospitals that do better than the average in terms of cost increases stand to gain, and hospitals that do less well than the average stand to lose in terms of reimbursement.

It should be obvious that these approaches are essentially designed to deal with relative inefficiency rather than with inflation.* That is not to say that such approaches do not have merit—they do—but rather to indicate that in general the potential is limited to eliminating technical inefficiency, which could of course be of a significant order of magnitude. The apparent rate of inflation in the hospital sector would be moderated if such incentive reimbursement were to lead to an increase in the average level of technical efficiency.

Among the incentive-reimbursement proposals, one that has attracted

*Unless it is held that technical inefficiency has increased over time, leading to inflation.

interest is prospective budgeting. There are many variations on the theme, but the principle involves the establishment of prospective budgets that provide the basis for prospective rates. The incentive component in prospective budgeting and rate setting is the chance for an institution to gain or lose according to whether it underruns or overruns the prospective budget negotiated with its third-party payer. It is likely that prospective budgeting has its greatest potential in the context of eliminating relative inefficiency. Prospective budgeting, however, implicitly assumes some negotiation with an outside review or audit agency. The negotiation process can include efforts to affect demand, the expansion of facilities and services, and relative efficiency. Hence, prospective budgeting has the same potential for controlling costs as any incentive-reimbursement approach directed specifically at any or all of these areas.

Although incentive reimbursement represents a broad spectrum of activities, its essence is to provide incentives to contain costs. Either positive or negative inducements can be applied, and any factor that affects cost or cost inflation can be the subject of incentive reimbursement. In practice, however, negative incentives are more likely to affect the outcome and, in general, incentive reimbursement alone is more likely to have an impact on relative inefficiency. Incentive reimbursement is least likely to affect hospital cost inflation through controlling demand, and more likely to affect cost inflation, when negative incentives are used in conjunction with areawide planning and certification of need to control the expansion of facilities and services.

While a theoretical distinction can be made between negative incentives and controls, rate regulation is not far removed from negative incentives in practice. If the inflation of hospital costs approximates the process that was outlined in the previous section, then rate regulation would seem to have the potential to control hospital inflation. If rates are controlled, then revenues are controlled. If revenues are not available, then there is a real constraint on the ability of hospitals to add to the quality and complexity of the scope of services provided. Rate regulation should moderate the rate of inflation. What evidence is there of the impact of rate regulation on the inflation process under the Economic Stabilization Program?

RECENT PRICE TRENDS

Some preliminary and tentative indication of the impact that rate regulation might have on hospital cost inflation can be inferred from the data in Tables 8 and 9. The data for 1969 and 1970 reflect the trends

TABLE 8 Average Annual Percentage Increases in Prices, Costs, and Real Inputs in Nonfederal Short-Term General Hospitals, 1969-1972

	Average Annual Increases (%)			
	1969	1970	1971	1972
Consumer Price Index	5.4	5.9	4.3	3.3
Hospital daily service charge	13.4	12.9	12.2	6.6
Average cost per patient day	14.1	15.7	13.9	14.0
Average cost per admission	13.2	13.7	11.1	11.7
Personnel per patient day	2.6	3.9	3.4	3.0
Nonlabor inputs per patient day[a]	9.8	11.0	9.5	14.2
Real inputs per patient day[a]	6.2	7.4	5.6	6.5

SOURCE: Consumer Price Index and hospital daily service charge, *in* Consumer Price Index. Washington, D.C., Bureau of Labor Statistics; Average cost data and personnel data, *in* Hospital Statistics 1972. Chicago, American Hospital Association.
[a]See Table 6.

TABLE 9 Average Net Revenues per Year in Nonfederal Short-Term General Hospitals, 1969-1972

	1969	1970	1971	1972
Net revenue: total revenue	3.2	2.7	2.7	1.9
Net revenue: plant assets	3.2	2.8	3.0	2.1

SOURCE: Hospitals (Guide Issue), 1970-1971; Hospital Statistics 1971-1972. Chicago, American Hospital Association.

that prevailed in the latter part of the 1960s, and should serve as a convenient base of reference for the trends under rate regulation as imposed by the Economic Stabilization Program. In fact, the impact of rate regulation must be inferred from the data for 1971 and 1972.

The Economic Stabilization Program was initiated on August 15, 1971, with a 90-day freeze on prices, wages, salaries, and rents. Thus, the 1971 data in Tables 8 and 9 can be used to infer the probable impact of Phase I, which was in effect for only part of the year. It would appear that the controls did have an impact in 1971 on hospital prices and on the cost of hospital inputs, but probably did not have a significant impact on the root cause of inflation. The rate of increase of hospital prices as measured by the daily service charge was lowered somewhat in 1971, as was the rate of increase of hospital costs measured by either the average cost per patient day or average cost per admission. However, the effect on input costs was probably slightly greater and the net effect on hospital revenues may well have been favorable. Hospital net revenues were as high or higher in 1971 than they had been in 1970.*

Phase II of the Economic Stabilization Program covered the period from November 1971 through January 1973 and, hence, the 1972 data in Tables 8 and 9 can be used to infer the probable impact of Phase II, which was in effect for the entire year.† Rate regulation under the program does seem to have had a real impact on the rate of increase of hospital prices and on the potential for hospital cost inflation. The rate of increase of prices was slowed considerably; the annual percentage increase in the daily service charge of 6.6 percent was the lowest rate of increase since 1965. The rate of increase of hospital costs, however, was not lower in 1972 than it had been in 1971; both the average cost per patient day and per admission were slightly higher in 1972 than in 1971. The real impact of the controls was translated into a reduction in the net revenues of hospitals in 1972. The net revenue ratios of short-term general hospitals were lower in 1972 than they had been in any year since 1964. If the inflation of hospital costs does in fact approximate the process outlined above, then the Economic Stabilization Program would seem to have had a real impact. Apparently by controlling rates in 1972, the program controlled net revenues in 1972. If net revenues are not available, there is a real constraint on the ability of hospitals to add facilities and services that enhance quality and expand complexity with a consequent increase in the cost of production.

The data in Table 8 also serve to point up the lag between the imposition of controls and the eventual moderation of inflation that should be expected. Expansion is not instantaneous. The decision-making process undoubtedly is time consuming. The increased demand and inflation in earlier years provided net revenues that funded expansion with cost consequences in later years. One would expect that the lower net revenues in 1972 would inhibit expansion in 1973 and later, with concomitant cost consequences in still later years.‡ It is probably too

*The data indicate that the rate of increase of prices peaked in 1969, while the rate of increase of costs peaked in 1970, and suggest that at least a word of caution is in order concerning any inferences that might be drawn. There is not sufficient evidence in these aggregate data to separate the effect of Phase I on net revenues from the effect of the differential rates of increase of prices and costs prior to August 15, 1971. In fact, the level of demand is a major missing piece of information in this analysis of Phase I and in the analysis of Phase II that follows. The analysis implicitly assumes no significant change in demand.

†As those familiar with hospital statistics will recognize, data are usually for the year ending September 30 or for the fiscal year closest to that date and, hence, the 1972 data may well reflect the impact of Phase I, as well as Phase II. Further, it is quite likely that the data for 1971 were affected little by Phase I.

‡It might be tempting to ascribe the downward trend in the personnel per patient day to the controls and draw the obvious conclusion. Such may be the case, but it is really too soon to have much confidence in such limited evidence.

soon to draw any definitive conclusions concerning the eventual impact of the Economic Stabilization Program. The reflections in this section must be viewed in the proper perspective. The data provide some indication of the impact of rate regulation on hospital cost inflation, but these are preliminary and tentative—even somewhat speculative.

CONCLUSIONS

Hospital cost inflation is not a recent problem, but represents a phenomenon of long standing that has intensified in recent years. A reflection on long-term price trends in the context of the structure of the hospital sector and behavioral patterns associated with nonprofit hospitals suggests that the process of inflation is best explained as demand-induced inflation. Higher real incomes, population growth, a change in population mix, and most especially an increase in both private and public insurance coverage have led to an increase in the demand for hospital care. The increase in demand has induced a supply response, but part of the supply response has taken the form of an increase in quality and an increase in the complexity of the scope of services offered with a consequent increase in the cost of hospital care over time.

It is possible to contain hospital cost inflation. If the inflation process can be approximated as it has been above, then incentive reimbursement and, particularly, rate regulation have a distinct potential for moderating hospital cost inflation. The reflections on these controls, however, would be less than complete without an emphasis on the delicate balance that must be struck between controlling costs that are inappropriate and undesirable to restrain increased quantities of both labor and nonlabor inputs per patient, without inhibiting increases that are appropriate and desirable. In effect, care must be given lest the controls are too effective.

What is implied, of course, is that price controls, incentive-reimbursement mechanisms, and rate regulation must be applied in conjunction with other policy instruments. Incentive reimbursement integrated with areawide planning and certification of need represent one such development in this context. The special exception procedure built into Phase IV enabling the Cost of Living Council to approve additional revenues where there is a demonstrated community need for new facilities and services suggests that current price-control policy has evolved with some concern for an appropriate balance.

REFERENCES AND NOTES

1. Feldstein M: The Rising Cost of Hospital Care. Information Resources Press, 1971; Hospital cost inflation: A study of nonprofit price dynamics. Am Econ Rev pp 853–872 (December 1971); Davis K: Hospital costs and the Medicare program. Soc Secur Bull pp 18–36 (August 1973).
2. See for example: Davis K: Economic theories of behavior in nonprofit private hospitals. Econ Bus Bull, pp 1–13 (Winter 1972); Feldstein M: Hospital cost inflation: A study of nonprofit price dynamics, *op. cit.;* Lee ML: A conspicuous production theory of hospital behavior. Southern Econ J, pp 48–58 (July 1971); Newhouse J: Toward a theory of nonprofit institutions: An economic model of a hospital. Am Econ Rev, pp 64–74 (March 1970); and Pauly M, Redisch M: The not-for-profit hospitals as a physicians' cooperative. Am Econ Rev, pp 87–100 (March 1973).

HAROLD COHEN, Ph.D.
Health Services Cost Review Commission
Department of Health and Mental Hygiene, State of Maryland

State Rate Regulation

Issues involved in state rate regulation of health care providers include whether rate regulation should be left to the market; which providers, if any, to regulate; how the rate-setting body should be organized, and how it will relate organizationally to other state agencies regulating health providers; and how a rate-regulating body should set rates. This essay centers more on rate level and rate structure than on the process of rate setting, although that also contains problems. Other issues discussed briefly are budgeting method, data quality, and medical staff privileges. My principal remarks will concern organization and rate-setting methodology and some of the approaches the Maryland Health Services Cost Review Commission has taken or is likely to take in dealing with these matters.

The Health Services Cost Review Commission (HSCRC) was established by the 1971 Maryland General Assembly. The commission was given specific responsibilities with various commencement dates and certain powers to achieve those responsibilities.

The facilities the commission regulates are hospitals and related institutions. *Related institutions* is a term in law and does not mean what it might appear to mean on the basis of common usage. *Related institutions* is defined in Section 556 of the Maryland Code and basically covers nursing homes and care homes. Some treatment centers for alcoholics also are included.

The first commission responsibility is public disclosure of the financial position of these institutions. This responsibility began the day the commission was appointed, July 1, 1971. The second main area of responsibility concerns the relationship between costs, services, and charges. The commission must certify that total costs are reasonably related to total services offered, that aggregate rates are set in reasonable relationship to aggregate costs, and that rates are set equitably without undue discrimination. These responsibilities, as of now, begin July 1, 1974, for hospitals and July 1, 1975, for related institutions.

The commission has certain powers to meet these responsibilities. It could collect accounting records (i.e., it has subpoena power) and hold public hearings as of July 1, 1971. A uniform accounting and reporting system has been developed for hospitals and related institutions. These institutions, by law, had to adopt the appropriate system at the start of their fiscal year beginning on or after April 1, 1973. As a part of its power to ensure meaningful disclosure and to assure that costs, rates, and services provided are reasonably related; HSCRC can require full or partial audit and verification by independent certified public accountants.

The main issue for today's discussion is the Maryland law, which, in effect, makes the covered institutions public utilities. Beginning July 1, 1974, for hospitals and July 1, 1975, for related institutions, the commission shall have the power to carry out investigations so that it may "assure all purchasers of health care institutions that the total cost of the institutions are reasonably related to the total services offered . . . that . . . aggregate rates are reasonably related to . . . aggregate costs . . . and that rates are set equitably among all purchasers or classes of purchasers of services without undue discrimination or preference."

As mentioned earlier, the enabling legislation specifically spells out the commission's rate-setting powers (from Section 568U of Article 43 of the Annotated Code of Maryland):

> In order to properly discharge these obligations, the Commission shall have full power to review and approve the reasonableness of rates established or requested by any institution subject to the provisions of this subtitle. No institution shall charge for services at a rate other than those established in accordance with the procedures established hereunder.
>
> In the interest of promoting the most efficient and effective use of health care institutional service, the Commission may promote and approve alternative methods of rate determination and payment of an experimental nature that may be in the public interest and consistent with the purposes of this subtitle.

The rates the commission sets are thus both maxima and minima.

That "hospitals and nursing homes" is currently Maryland's legal answer concerning which providers should be regulated, does not make it a correct or precise answer. The power to regulate is that of controlling the institution's rates. This leaves HSCRC in an uncertain position with regard to hospital-based physicians, including pathologists, radiologists, and anesthesiologists. Many of these physicians have contracts with hospitals by which they receive a percentage of the gross or net receipts of their departments. By controlling departmental rates, the state is, in effect, regulating the per-unit revenues of those physicians. Those hospital-based physicians who bill directly, however, would not be subject to such regulation.

The commission feels that the way in which such physicians bill is a matter of form rather than substance and that their rates should be regulated, regardless. These specialists are not selected by the patient, but rather by the hospital and its medical staff. Once a patient enters the hospital, he has no choice of pathologist; nor is he likely to ever meet the one he pays. Consumers can not shop among these specialists if they do not like their rates; there is usually only one group with privileges at any hospital.

Under Medicare Part B, the federal government has not put nearly as much pressure on physicians as it has on hospitals under Part A, but there are fewer dollars spent under Part B. Percentage of revenue contracts in radiology and pathology are linked with internal rate structures by which losses in obstetrics and emergency rooms, for instance, are subsidized by profits in radiology and pathology. If a hospital has a 30 percent of gross contract, it could shift $150,000 revenue out of, say, radiology; raise obstetrical rates by $150,000; and be just as well off. That is one of the procedures the commission's rate structure will facilitate, but more on that later.

Other states would do well to write their statutes so that hospital-based physicians are covered. The commission tried, during the 1973 session of the Maryland legislature, to amend the definition of hospital institutional services in such a way that hospital-based physicians would come under our jurisdiction, regardless of method of billing. The bill passed the Senate, but was killed in the House committee—largely, if not entirely, because of Maryland's medical society. The bill is being re-introduced this session with, hopefully, more success.

Another kind of provider not regulated by HSCRC is the Health Maintenance Organization (HMO). The Maryland commission has been subjected to pressure by both the Maryland Hospital Association and the Maryland Comprehensive Health Planning Agency but has indicated it does not want to regulate HMOs and would like to see that form of delivery given a chance to prove itself without interference. At a recent public hearing concerning a proposed moratorium on hospital beds in the Baltimore region, the commission gave testimony supporting the moratorium but urged that HMOs that could not work out satisfactory contracts with existing hospitals be exempted from the moratorium.[1]

Nursing homes with less than 30 beds have also been exempted administratively on the grounds that compliance costs would outweigh any potential gains and that the market will see that they cannot overcharge. It is quite possible that a larger cut-off size should have been chosen. There are 200 nursing homes in the state and that number may ensure a sufficient market protection. Before suggesting deregulation of nursing-home rates I would want more data. Preliminary examination of the disclosure information gathered indicates that 60–100-percent returns on equity in the industry (even with 100 percent Medicaid patients) is not unusual. I am, however, willing now to suggest that nursing homes not be subjected to certification-of-need laws if their rates are to be regulated on a target occupancy basis, as they will be in Maryland.

The second problem area mentioned is organization—both internal and with other state agencies regulating the relevant health providers. Since a public utility type approach is being assumed (and recommended), and since one of the major complaints concerning the public utility model is that regulatory agencies are co-opted by the industry they are established to regulate, the makeup and credibility of the regulatory body is quite important.

I propose an independent 3–7-member group financed at a level that enabled it to spend, perhaps, one day a week overseeing the job. The chairman might be a full-time commissioner of hospitals who did not have overall responsibility for either the state hospital system or the Medicaid program. Good rules of thumb are that one-third of the regulatory body, at most, should be allowed to have a financial interest in the industry and that a simple majority of affirmative votes be required to pass any motion.

The state of Maryland has not fully satisfied these suggestions. State law requires that four of the seven members "shall be persons who have no connection with the management or policy of any hospitals or related institutions." Further, state regulations that call for hearing subcommittees of three members require at least two of those to be the "unconnected" members. A further safeguard in the law is that "no action of the Commission shall be effective unless at least four (4) of its members concur therein" (Section J). This means that, even if the three "connected" persons found themselves in the majority at a commission meeting, they could not make any effective changes without some "unconnected" support.

More important is the nature of the membership. In my opinion, all have been representing the public and not any particular interest group. I feel they are doing a good job. The "unconnecteds" have strong opinions and are not the types to be dominated, and the "connecteds" provide expertise but are not stereotype AMA or hospital administrator individuals. As a consumer, I would feel satisfied.

Possibly a more serious problem in this area is HSCRC's current connection with the state Department of Health and Mental Hygiene. The enabling legislation states that the commission is "an independent commission functioning within the Department of Health and Mental Hygiene." The combined meaning of "independent" and "within" is unclear. The commission feels that independence is vital because the department is the largest provider of institutional health care (13 state mental, rehabilitation, and chronic hospitals), the second largest hospital payer, and the largest purchaser of care in related institutions (through Medicaid).[2] It can act independently of the department, but—if the department controls its budget and has veto power over its regulations, how independent will it appear to others?

The staff of the commission and the consultants working for it earn no money from providers. The main consultants are Haskins and Sells, which has no hospital audit clients in Maryland and after this year will no longer audit Blue Cross, and Hospital Cost Analysis Service, a nonprofit firm currently doing cost verifications for Medicare, Medicaid, and Blue Cross. A contrary example exists in New Jersey, where Blue Cross and Medicaid payment rates are presently set by the Advisory Committee to the Commissioners of Health and Insurance. Each hospital's budget is reviewed by one of six subcommittees, which has the responsibility of establishing a reasonable rate of payment based on these budget submissions. Each subcommittee consists of a hospital trustee, two hospital administrators, a physician, and a representative of the Department of Health.[3] In my view, this agency seems to have been captured by the industry it is supposed to regulate.

Unlike most regulatory agencies, such as the federal Civil Aeronautics Board and the Interstate Commerce Commission, which are subject to great industry pressure and little countervailing pressure from the millions of small individual consumers, an agency regulating rates of institutional health providers will attract close attention from Blue Cross, Medicare, Medicaid, and, perhaps, such other groups as the Health Insurance Council. HSCRC has invited Maryland Blue Cross to play a strong consumer advocacy role in its rate hearings, and Maryland Blue Cross is not a captive of Maryland's hospitals.

While there need be no direct administrative liaison with the licensing agency or with the Professional Standards Review Organization,[4] very close liaison must exist with the insurance commissioner, or whatever body regulates health insurance. The relationship among hospitals, insurance commissioner, Blue Cross, and Cost Commission is still developing in Maryland. It has led to some very interesting situations and, for Blue Cross especially, some potential and actual major problems.

As mentioned earlier, the rates the commission sets are both maxima and minima. This was written into the law by hospital interests, who felt that Blue Cross worked to their disadvantage, especially in the area of payment for bad debts. The effect of making a rate a minimum is that now Blue Cross essentially has to bargain with the commission for price concessions and cannot bargain individually with hospitals.

HSCRC has close liaison with the insurance department; one of the two deputy insurance commissioners is a member of the commission. According to an agreement, the commission sets the rates that Blue Cross pays hospitals and the insurance commissioner sets the rates that Blue Cross charges subscribers. There is, however, a timing problem that has, as yet, not been resolved.

The most important relationship is that with the Comprehensive Health Planning Agency, a group that controls certification of need. In Maryland this agency is separate from the commission and both are under the Department of Health and Mental Hygiene. I strongly believe that the two agencies should be one and that they should be independent of the department charged with running the state's provider facilities and the Medicaid program.[5] The same agency that sets supply (and thus generates capacity costs) and estimates demand should also set rates. HSCRC has good communication with CHP and performs financial feasibility analysis for proposed major projects, but that is not enough. A chronic problem with regulatory agencies is that in the past they have protected existing firms. With target occupancy rates set for the largely proprietary and relatively low capital intense nursing home industry, there should be no certification-of-need requirement.

The need for close liaison (or, preferably, identity) with CHP will become clearer in discussion of the rate level; but first I will outline the commission's system of setting prospective rates. This system has the incentive effect of creating a regulatory lag and also allows the rate-setting body to give fair warning that certain budget items will not be allowed in rates. There are two main differences between an appropriate rate level and that determined under present systems in other states. Currently there are classes of costs that are considered allowable and all costs in those categories are covered. The Maryland commission, however, identifies allowable cost categories, but—within those categories—recognizes only reasonable costs as reimbursable. The other difference is that, under the commission's system, costs will be estimated at target occupancies and divided by target occupancies, rather than achieved occupancies. Since some costs are fixed in the short run and since occupancy levels in Maryland are currently below achievable targets, this will result in lower rates. For example, by setting target occupancies in obstetrics around 70 percent, the commission can force certain hospitals to go to CHP and request permission to cease that service.

One major unresolved question is what relationship between fixed and variable costs would enable the commission to adjust experience to estimate what costs would have been at different occupancies and to adjust budgets to target figures. I am not enthusiastic about the fixed-variable ratio method proposed by the Cost of Living Council and prefer a more detailed budget analysis of what the fixed costs are in various departments.

One requirement for identifying reasonable cost is the ability to relate costs of one hospital with that of all the hospitals, or at least of some similar hospitals. The commission has developed a uniform accounting and reporting system that stipulates statistics for overhead and service areas.[6] It anticipates that the first round of rate setting will be a matter of establishing rates per statistic, such as per relative value unit in the operating room or per day for pediatrics. The latter rate, however, will be modified by an admissions charge, which will pick up those costs associated more with the number of cases than the number of patient days.

Another, and perhaps more controversial problem, is the rate of return for proprietary institutions. There is one proprietary general hospital and a few proprietary psychiatric hospitals in the state. Three more proprietary hospitals are being built, and the bulk of the nursing and care homes are proprietary institutions. HSCRC must set a fair rate of return—one that will attract the desired amount of capital into the industry. Clearly, the state and regional planning agencies would have an input into the adequacy of the facility supply in certain areas. The rate of return is based upon the riskiness of the investment and is a payment to encourage investors to put their money into health care facilities rather than alternative ventures or interest-bearing assets. The rate of return for nursing homes need not be uniform across the state. For example, there is currently an apparent surplus of applications for nursing homes in northwest Baltimore County and a shortage in southeast Baltimore City. This might indicate that currently achieved rates of return are higher than necessary to attract capital in the first location but too low to attract it in the second.

One practice that a return on equity system will eliminate is the current Medicaid markup on costs. Medicaid now pays cost plus 10 percent up to a maximum in the state. For example, one small home, which provided for no one but Medicaid patients, recently asked for a rate increase under Phase III and reported costs of $15.00 per day. It thus received $1.50 profit per patient day for the approximately 11,700 days consumed. This yielded a total profit of $17,500 on an equity of about $28,000. The firm, totally tax supported, was earning a 60 percent return on equity. The markup on expenses is about the most perverse payment method, as far as providing an incentive to efficiency, one can easily imagine.

Ideally, the rate level should not allow patients to subsidize losses in auxiliary institution enterprises. There are various expenses that should probably be covered from nonpatient sources. Such questions arise as—Should current patients pay the cost of training future nurses and doctors? Should patients pay for the costs generated by unused beds—for all excess capacity or a reasonable amount? Perhaps the community should pay for beds maintained as calamity insurance. The commission is in the position of saying whether the hospitals can charge patients. If the commission feels another revenue source is more appropriate (such as general taxes for charity care), it cannot require the other source to meet its obligations as determined by the commission. The hospital might suffer if the commission specified that patients could not be charged and then the other sources failed to materialize.

Another major issue is bad debts. Once a level of cost has been determined, and rates set related to those costs, what is to be done about bad debts? Medicare law says Medicare can not pay for the bad debts of noneligibles. Medicaid says in effect, "We pay our bills: why should we pay for someone else?" Blue Cross says the same. That approach leads to the conclusion that bad debts should be charged to patients who do not pay their bills. That is very equitable, but it is a joke as a policy. National health insurance will end the problem. An appropriate definition of medical indigency according to the Medicaid program would also solve the problem. Hospitals could go after the money owed them by anyone who did not pay but could afford to pay. This would lessen tremendously the quantitative effect of bad debts. The Maryland commission is a strong supporter of either of these solutions. In the meantime, bad debts are costs accrued by hospitals for which they are not receiving income and cause an undue drain on the provider.

Maryland Blue Cross does not pay any bad debts at present. Under the commission's rate-setting methodology covering those patients they do not insure, they will be expected to pay some. Since bad debts amount to about 5 percent of gross charges and originate from the 20 percent who self-pay, it means one in four self-pay patients do not pay their charges and the other three have to cover the whole bad debt load. A simplified example, which represents an average situation, might be as follows.

If the cost per day as defined by Blue Cross is \$80.00, and we assume that this is a proper cost and 80 percent of the patients' bills are settled on this basis; then, since only three quarters of the other 20 percent of patients pay their bills, the required average charge is \$106.70; that is

.80 (\$80) + .15 (\$106.70) = \$80 average received payment per day.

If bad debts were evenly distributed, then the required charge would be \$84.21; that is,

.95 (\$84.21) = \$80 average received.

Thus if bad debts were spread evenly over all patients, as in most retail operations, hospital rates (charges) could be reduced, in this example, by 21 percent; from \$106.70 to \$84.21.

Further, suppose actual cost were not \$80 as computed by definitions imposed on hospitals by the big payers, but actually \$82. Then charges would have to be \$120.00; that is,

.80 (\$80) + .15 (\$120) = \$82 average received.

The \$2 disallowance results in an increase of \$13.30 in the required charges. Here, an average rate might be \$86.32; that is,

.95 (\$86.32) = \$82 average received.

In this instance, a uniform redefinition of cost and spread of bad debts would reduce rates 28 percent, from \$120.00 to \$86.32. The opposite effect would occur if actual cost were below cost as defined by Blue Cross. One problem that aggravates the importance of these charges is that it is the charges, or at least some of them, that are reflected in the cost of living measures. Another problem is that self-pay patients are often hard working people earning slightly too much to qualify for Medicaid and without hospitalization insurance; they are not usually the wealthy, self-insured individuals.

This explains at least in part the inclusion of the minimum rate aspect of commission-established rates. An important thing to remember is that we are talking about prospective rate setting. The expenses we discussed are those predicted for a specific occupancy rate during the forthcoming year. The rate level should be designed to allow the hospital to cover its costs as they would be generated at an occupancy rate representing a reasonably effective use of the facility. The remaining question is how to generate the required revenue; this is the problem of rate structure.

RATE STRUCTURE

The main, if not the only legal, requirement of the rate structure is that rates be "set equitably among all purchasers or classes of purchasers of services without undue discrimination or preference" (Section U). This phrase includes two aspects, neither of which is extremely clear. "Classes of purchasers of services," I feel, should apply both to distinctions as to groups of purchasers divided according to source of revenue (e.g., Blue Cross, Medicaid, Medicare) and as to types of services bought.

We have not discussed the current rate structure as to type of service. In many hospitals, revenues from radiology, pathology, pharmacy, and the like subsidize losses in such departments as obstetrics and emergency room. Three reasons for this are (1) high bad debts in the latter areas; (2) Blue Cross paying charges for covered outpatients' diagnostic services, but only cost for inpatient services; and (3) low occupancy in maternity, coupled with state laws that keep some other patients out of the empty maternity beds.

The commission has the power to redesign the rate schedule to preclude this kind of internal cross-subsidization. There is no equitable reason why inpatients should be held financially accountable for the cost of services provided clinic, obstetric, and emergency room patients who do not pay their bills.

The phrase "undue discrimination" means, at a minimum, that no customer or class of customer is charged less than the differential (added) cost the institution incurs in serving them. Perhaps, also, no group should be charged more than the long-run average cost of providing the service it is buying (cost includes a profit return for risk). Other questions to be considered here are the types of experiments to use. Should there be more hospitals on an all-inclusive rate? Should there be a charge based on diagnosis—so many dollars for an uncomplicated tonsillectomy?

The hardest task facing the commission is to develop incentives for efficiency. The people making decisions should be aware of the costs of those decisions and, where possible, bear the burden of the decisions. This includes putting more of a burden on physicians. Currently, if Blue Cross determines that a patient was hospitalized for diagnostic purposes, Blue Cross will not pay the hospital bill but Blue Shield (still physician-dominated) will pay the doctor's bill. Perhaps the physician should be responsible for the hospital's bill.

Prospective rate setting also automatically provides a six month or one year regulatory lag. For example, if costs were reduced during the year, the hospital could be allowed to keep the full savings. Also, future rates might leave some of those savings with the hospital. Hospitals could keep some of the funds generated if they lowered their costs and absorbed some of the losses incurred by exceeding projected costs. A recently proposed Blue Cross contract would have allowed the hospital to retain 20 percent of cost below and absorb 80 percent of cost above some mutually agreed upon target. The insurance commissioner wanted to see a limit to the percent of bad debts Blue Cross could pay, and the hospitals refused such a limitation. The insurance commissioner, therefore, denied approval of the contract.

There will be a strong incentive to achieve high levels of occupancy. Under the current system, for 80 percent of a hospital's inpatients there is no incentive to schedule effectively. Costs are divided by achieved occupancy, so lower occupancy simply means higher settlement rates. This pressure will be countervailed by an active PSRO.

A final area of cost savings is in the area of reports and audits. Hospitals now make reports for all three payers. The commission will consolidate this function by certifying to each payer that charges reflect cost.

As an example of misplaced burdens and how the system works, consider Medicare deliberating whether or not to have the hospitals adopt one additional report form. Assume this form will impose $1,000 per hospital in compliance costs. The national compliance cost would be about $6 million, but Medicare rules call for that cost to be spread over all patients. Assuming 20 percent of patients to be Medicare, the added cost to Medicare would be $1.2 million. Their decision rule could thus be: "If this information is worth more than $1.2 million, adopt the requirement." If the return to Medicare was, say, $2 million, the report would be adopted even though its true cost was three-times its benefit.

Part of all compliance costs are allocated to self-pay patients who cause none of them. The major problem is efficiency rather than equity. For example, if a plan pays 20 percent of $4 million rather than 25 percent of $1 million, it is the dollar volume difference rather than the percentage difference that causes the biggest problem. By moving toward prospective rates, including a return on equity, and away from actual expenses and markups on expenses, the rewards will be more properly structured, but only if these rates are based upon reasonable expenses and effective utilization.

Three final problems arise in this area of how to finance the regulating agency, physician privileges, and hospital trustee conflicts of interest. I believe the regulatory agency should be financed by a charge on the institutions but that this should not be a percentage of gross due to the up-front conflict of interest. A regulatory charge might best be included in the admission charge. HSCRC is budgeted through general tax funds and our budget is reviewed first by the Department of Health and Mental Hygiene, which is the largest provider of institutional health care, the largest purchaser of nursing home care, and the third largest purchaser of hospital care in Maryland. Those conflicts can and have hurt our credibility.

I strongly believe that successful elimination of excess duplication requires more open privileges. Currently, there are 13 emergency rooms in Baltimore open on weekends because doctors want to meet their patients at the emergency room but only have privileges at one or two hospitals. If you try to eliminate a service in a circumstance that doctors cannot easily provide the service elsewhere, there will be a terrible fight. Here HSCRC is trying to help the administrators and trustees withstand medical staff pressure. We have a bill in the 1974 Maryland legislature to open privileges to all licensed or board-certified physicians.

Trustees are politically powerful individuals. As a group, they represent most of the banking and construction interests. Many lawyers and legislators are also on boards, including the two legislators who introduced our enabling legislation (which had strong industry support, remember).

The Washington Post ran an interesting series of articles, which raised interest in this in Maryland. As a result, the legislature passed a law requiring that trustees who are owners or beneficial owners of 3 percent of a firm that gets more than $10,000 worth of business from his hospital must report the business connection and the amount of business to the commission. We have developed proposed regulations to adopt that law and they have generated interest from many other states.

The existence of such relationships does not necessarily indicate that the hospital is being victimized, but implies a possibility of easier negotiations between trustee and hospital. Many hospitals may keep excess amounts of money in non-interest-bearing accounts in trustees' banks. HSCRC will be studying the potential problem with that arrangement. Meanwhile, there have been some trustee resignations and complaints. The commission received a letter from a hospital trustee who stated that he was the hospital's radiologist and had a contract with the hospital giving him 35 percent of the gross in his department. He wondered if that could be a conflict of interest. Making the public aware of such relationships—and everything our commission collects is public—may have some interesting consequences.

In conclusion, there are still many unsolved issues in how to apply the utility regulation model to hospitals and nursing homes, but it offers potential solutions to major problems if handled correctly. I do not believe every state should adopt this approach until it has been given a chance to prove itself.

REFERENCES AND NOTES

1. Testimony of Health Services Cost Review Commission before Regional Planning Council.
2. HSCRC: Second Annual Report to Governor.
3. Correspondence with New Jersey rate reviewer.
4. There is an active admissions review program for all Medicaid patients in Maryland. This is run by a foundation set up by Maryland Medical Society.
5. See the Commission's Second Annual Report.
6. HSCRC: Uniform Accounting and Reporting System for Hospitals, April 1, 1973.

V

Regulation of Payment to Physicians

The manner in which the non-institutional practitioner is reimbursed for health care services to ambulatory patients has an effect on both the utilization and cost of the services. In this section, Uwe E. Reinhardt surveys some alternative arrangements and their probable consequences. He also examines in detail the implications that a fee-for-service mechanism would have if incorporated into a national health insurance plan, and makes some recommendations for using fee schedules to improve the efficiency of the system.

A panel discussion of the Reinhardt concepts was conducted by Marvin Shapiro, M.D., practicing physician and chairman of the board of trustees, California Blue Shield; Irwin Wolkstein, deputy director for program policy, Bureau of Health Insurance, Social Security Administration; Michael Halberstam, M.D., practicing physician, Washington, D.C.

The final paper is an overview of the other conference papers and discussions, as seen by Jonathan Spivak, Washington, D.C., health affairs reporter for The Wall Street Journal.

UWE E. REINHARDT, Ph.D.
Assistant Professor of Economics
and
Woodrow Wilson School of Public and International Affairs, Princeton University

Alternative Methods of Reimbursing Non-institutional Providers of Health Services

In any area of economic activity involving the transfer of goods or services from producers to consumers, the financial arrangement accompanying that transfer tends to exert a strong influence on the real resource costs of the product and on the financial resources transferred from consumers to producers. Embedded in the financial arrangement is a variety of economic incentives to which both consumers and producers respond, typically in predictable fashion. This very predictability furnishes the cornerstone of modern economic theory.

That standard economic principles can safely be grafted onto the markets for watermelons, bread, furniture, automobile repairs, or even purchased affection is widely taken for granted. By their own admission, the producers of such commodities are "in it mainly for the money." Consumers, on the other hand, are generally capable of assessing the quality of such products and of choosing among them with the detachment of the rational *homo oeconomicus.* The power of pecuniary incentives in that context seems self-evident.

The question is whether standard economic theory is at all helpful in the analysis of professional services or, to put it another way, whether an economist ought to be invited to speak on the topic before this audience. This is not a rhetorical question. Among non-economists, the economist's attempt to formulate rigorous models of health care delivery is not uncommonly met with some bemusement, or even with some irritation. The bemusement may be triggered by the image of a critically injured patient consuming his or her last energy in the complex hedonistic calculus that culminates in what economists call the "price-elasticity of the demand for medical care." Some irritation may be found among physicians who, as other professionals, pride themselves on a relentless dedication to the substance of their profession—the alleviation or prevention of human suffering—and who deem the conduct of their practice to be impervious to pecuniary incentives. (This image of selfless dedication, incidentally, is one that virtually all professionals seek to instill among the laity, often with generous help from the information media. Can one imagine, for example, a Perry Mason ever billing his clients, or a Marcus Welby ever reading *Medical Economics* and worrying about his collection ratio?)

In this essay, the behavioral model of the classical *homo oeconomicus* is unabashedly grafted onto modern medical practice. In so doing, I do not assert that the consumer's demand for virtually all types of health care is fairly sensitive to price, nor suggest that physicians practice medicine solely for the money, but merely that a significant number of medical services are not unlike ordinary commodities and that their consumption can be analyzed with conventional consumer-choice theory. Similarly, it is postulated that pecuniary gain is one of a number of professional objectives pursued by the typical physician and that, if not all of the professional acts of physicians in this country are responsive to economic stimuli, a number of them nevertheless are. The implicit assumption, in other words, is that the conduct of medical practices is sensitive to economic incentives at the margin, and that this margin is sufficiently significant to be of interest to the formulators of the nation's health policy.

The remainder of this essay falls into two parts. The first is a broad survey of alternative financial arrangements that may accompany the delivery of ambulatory health care, and of the effects these arrangements are likely to have on the per capita utilization of health services and on the production costs of these services. The second is more narrowly focused on the economic implications of fee-for-service reimbursement. This closer look at one of many conceivable payment systems is offered on the premise that, whatever form national health insurance in this country ultimately will take, it is likely to accommodate the medical profession's penchant for fee-for-service reimbursement.

ALTERNATIVE FINANCIAL ARRANGEMENTS IN HEALTH CARE DELIVERY[1]

Although the financial arrangements accompanying the delivery of health care can take on a myriad of specific forms, for analytic purposes they can be sorted into a few distinct types. Table 1 presents a sorting that seems relevant for present purposes. The vertical and horizontal dimensions of the table are thought to represent the direct financial impact the consumers and providers of health services experience each time a unit of medical service passes between them. These direct costs or benefits will be referred to also as *marginal net benefits or costs.* A negative designation is interpreted as a monetary net cost, a positive one as a monetary net benefit. Psychic costs or benefits are left out of the picture.

Systems under which patients either do not have any health insurance coverage at all or under which they face significant coinsurance rates fall somewhere in column A of Table 1. Systems under which patients have complete first-dollar insurance coverage correspond to column B.[2] Column C might strike one as purely hypothetical, were it not for the fact that in some countries, e.g., West Germany, it is possible to obtain certain sick benefits contingent on the consumption of physician care.

On the provider side, the traditional fee-for-service systems fall into row C of the table. Systems under which individual providers are reimbursed automatically on a full average cost basis, or under which phy-

TABLE 1 Alternative Financial Arrangements in Health Care Delivery

Marginal Financial Impact on Providers Each Time a Service Is Rendered	Marginal Financial Impact on Consumer Each Time a Service Is Received		
	A. Negative	B. Zero	C. Positive
C. Positive	CA (Fee-for-service without insurance or high co-insurance)	CB (First-dollar insurance coverage with fee-for-service reimbursement)	CC –
B. Zero	BA (An outpatient department in a hospital charging patients a fee)	BB (A national health service as, for example, in the Soviet Union)	BC –
A. Negative	AA (Prepayment with some utilization fees)	AB (Prepayment without utilization fees–HMOs)	AC –

sicians receive a salary based on seniority rather than some rate of activity, fall into row B. Finally, systems under which providers deliver health care against prepayment of a prepaid annual capitation fee correspond to row A.[3,4]

The financial arrangements in Table 1 can affect the cost of health maintenance in two distinct ways. First, they may directly affect the overall level and mix of the per capita utilization of medical services. Second, they may influence the relative efficiency—and hence the real resource costs—with which they are produced.

Financial Incentives and the Utilization of Health Services

According to the familiar Law of Demand, the quantity demanded of almost any good or service per unit of time tends to vary inversely with its price, other things being equal. Few students of the health care sector today would argue that this law does not apply also to the broad category of services lumped together under the name *health care*, even if the demand for certain acute procedures (e.g., the setting of a broken leg or abdominal surgery) is totally insensitive to price. What is not known accurately is precisely how sensitive the demand for health care is to price (i.e., the so-called "price elasticity of demand"). Empirical research on the question has generally pointed to a rather low price sensitivity. It would be more revealing, however, to estimate these price elasticities for particular procedures. One suspects *a priori* that the price sensitivity of elective procedures—e.g., routine visits to the physician's office and preventive care—may be quite high. But whatever the actual case may be, it is undoubtedly safe to advance the proposition that, other things being equal, consumers in cells CB, BB, and AB of Table 1 will tend to consume more in total medical services than will consumers in cells CA, BA, or AA.

As a first approximation it is reasonable to suppose that a provider whose income or profit increases directly in proportion with the number of services he renders (row A of Table 1) would seek to maximize the number of services rendered per unit of time (or per unit of his time). Conversely, providers whose income varies inversely with the number of services rendered per unit of time may be expected to minimize the delivery of services subject, of course, to certain legal, ethical, or market constraints. In conventional markets, this motivation is found perfectly acceptable. It is assumed that consumers in that context are able to fend for themselves and effectively check any penchant for over- or undersupply.

In the professional services sector, however, the consumer's role in the formulation of his or her demand is typically more limited. Strictly speaking, the consumer exercises full autonomy only in the decision of whether or not to contact that sector. Once the contact is made, a professional typically takes on the role of "management consultant," counseling the consumer in the management of his or her legal, financial, pedagogic, or medical affairs. Although it would be going too far to assert that the individual consumer is completely passive in the formulation of the demand for the professional's services, much of the responsibility for formulating that demand is typically delegated to the professional. The latter is therefore active on both sides of the market, so to speak: He is at once the consumer's agent *and* one of the suppliers who meets the demand partially formulated by him as the consumer's agent.

The absence of complete independence between supply and demand in the market for professional services obviously engenders some awkward moral problems. There is, after all, the possibility that the influence professionals exert over the demand for their services is sensitive to the financial incentives they face. Perhaps for that reason the eighteenth century philosopher David Hume proposed that "every man should be paid in proportion to the trust reposed in him and to the power which he enjoys,"[5] a proposition that Adam Smith[6] subsequently elaborated thusly:

> We trust our health to the physician; our fortune and sometimes our life and reputation to the lawyer and attorney. Such confidence could not be safely reposed in people of a very mean and low condition. Their reward must be such, therefore, as may give them that rank in society which so important a trust requires.

In as genteel a way as is possible, Adam Smith suggests here that moral sentiments are a "luxury good" of which more will be consumed as income rises. The obvious implication is that to pay a professional a niggardly wage is to tempt him or her, and that to do so may have dire consequences indeed. In one of his recent papers, Mark Pauly[7] has incorporated this notion quite formally into a model of physician behavior. In that model the physician's own subjective interpretations of the medical code of ethics is thought to become ever more "liberal" as the difficulty of earning a satisfactory income mounts.

Adam Smith suggests how much a professional health care provider should be paid, but not in what manner. George Bernard Shaw,[8] never one to mince words, is more to the point in his famous lament:

> That any nation, having observed that you could provide for the supply of bread by giving bakers a pecuniary interest in baking for you, should go on to give a surgeon

a pecuniary interest in cutting off your leg, is enough to make one despair of political humanity.

Shaw is referring here to fee-for-service reimbursement (row C of Table 1). It has to be conceded that, in its economic dimensions at least, that reimbursement mode makes the doctor–patient relationship a perfect analogue of the agent–client relationship usually found in the repair of automobiles (or of consumer durables in general), and in the life insurance business. In view of the often unsavory reputations of these lines of business, physicians will most probably object to this analogy. They may argue, for example, that different occupations are bound by different codes of ethics and that the medical code is one of the strictest of its kind. Furthermore, physicians can point to the fact that the typical physician in this country is far too busy to have to compromise his professional ethics for the sake of pecuniary gain. I do not take issue with these propositions. The point is that, regardless of the presence or absence of a strict code of ethics and regardless of current supply conditions, a latent conflict of economic interest does exist under systems in row C, at least in principle, and the mere existence of a potential conflict of interest is warrant for some concern.

First, while the medical code of ethics is indeed lofty in spirit and strict in language, its enforcement need not be and apparently has not been commensurately strict. I know of no profession that has been notably successful in self-regulation. Second, the fact that the currently taut supply of physicians has served to protect the application of medical science from the pressure of pecuniary incentives is no assurance that this independence would survive conditions of relative excess supply, conditions that seem to be in the offing in this country. Third, and most important, in postulating the likelihood of physician-induced demand for physician services, one need not even appeal to baser economic motives or an erosion of moral sentiments; the application of medical science to human illness is a sufficiently imprecise enterprise to permit great leeway in practice patterns even on purely medical grounds. Furthermore, a good part of medical practice involves decision making on the basis of empirical information concerning the patient's health status and it can rightly be held that "the more information the better." Since both patients and physicians have long been conditioned to view the resource-intensity of medical treatment as an important index of its quality, it is only reasonable to assume that, where physicians are in ample supply, even marginally beneficial diagnostic or therapeutic procedures will be performed, and that the normal physician–patient encounter will be lengthened to absorb the available physician time.

This development is all the more probable where patients are covered by health insurance and many of them do not directly or indirectly bear the full cost of their own treatment. In short, there is no reason to suppose that medical practice is immune from a quite innocent application of Parkinson's Law. (It may be argued, of course, that any physician-induced increase in the "demand" for physician services is apt to increase also the quality of the treatment being dispensed, even if the extra services are not absolutely necessary. If one excepts from this assertion elective surgery, this may be a valid point and one an economist is not equipped to dispute. An economist can point out, however, that the added quality comes at a price, and that it is pertinent always to ask whether the quality so added is worth that price.)

As noted above, the argument that the rate at which physicians prescribe the use of their services is positively related to the marginal remuneration they earn on them is not novel.[9] In all fairness, however, it must be added that the empirical evidence bearing on this hypothesis is far from conclusive. This lack of conclusive evidence may indicate either that the medical code of ethics is indeed sufficiently strong to render the alleged conflict of interest ineffective at all times, or that the physician supply in recent years has been sufficiently taut to render the conflict temporarily ineffective. In any event, at this point one is justified only in offering the more circumspect proposition that under arrangements falling into row C of Table 1, providers are less likely to discourage any over-utilization of health services—or that they are more likely to apply complex and costly treatments in the management of a particular disease—than they would be under arrangements in rows B or A. Alternatively, it may be assumed that under arrangements in row A, providers of health care are more likely to be conservative in prescribing or applying medical services to the treatment of a medical condition than they would be under arrangements in rows B or C.

One further point needs to be raised in connection with the provider side. So far the discussion has proceeded on the implicit assumption that the "non-institutional provider" under consideration is the attending physician himself. One can imagine systems, however, in which the provider is some organization—e.g., an HMO or a medical foundation—which in turn employs the attending physician or procures the services rendered to patients by subcontracting with a physician. In principle it is possible that the provider renders services to patients on a fee-for-service basis while employing the physician on a salaried basis. Some outpatient visits in hospitals are delivered under this arrangement. Alternatively, the provider may render services against prepaid capitation fees while reimbursing the individual physician on a fee-for-service basis (as is the case under a medical foundation). In either case, the individual physician will remain the key element in the determination of health-services utilization, although the economic incentives he faces as an individual may not coincide with those of the "provider." It is difficult to predict just what effect the financial arrangement between providers and consumers would have on utilization rates under these circumstances. Much would depend on the extent of control the provider organization can exercise over the attending physician. A rigorous analysis of the organizational variants feasible in such cases lies beyond the scope of this essay. At this point it suffices to note that there may occasionally be a conflict between the incentives faced by the individual physicians and by non-institutional providers of care. For the moment, it is pretended that these incentives always coincide.

The preceding behavioral hypotheses permit one to make some broad generalizations concerning the utilization patterns likely to obtain under the various financial arrangements in Table 1. In making these predictions, it is analytically convenient to assume initially that the technology of health care production (and hence the resource costs per unit of service) is the same under all financial arrangements. That assumption will be relaxed in due course.

Under arrangements CA and AB, the financial incentives faced by consumers and providers work in opposite directions. Cell CA is representative of the traditional fee-for-service system in the absence of health insurance or under an insurance scheme confronting consumers with significant coinsurance (as is the case under Part B of the Medicare program). Barring taut supply conditions, physicians under this system have an economic incentive to over-prescribe services. Their enthusiasm in this respect would, however, be tempered by the patient's resistance to high out-of-pocket costs. As noted above, how strong the incentive to over-prescribe is, in fact, and how strong the patient's resistance to such a tendency might be, is as yet an open question, and one on which more research would be desirable.

Cell AB is representative of prepayment for comprehensive care (as in Health Maintenance Organizations, HMOs) without utilization fees for individual services. Here the consumer is likely to demand more services per episode of illness (whether medically necessary or not) than the provider would like to deliver. Once again, one cannot predict with certainty whose preferences are likely to prevail. However, since a physician's power of persuasion in medical matters is typically strong, it seems reasonable to predict somewhat lower utilization rates under arrangement AB than would be observed under CA.[10] In fact, one cannot rule out the possibility that the utilization rates under this system will be unduly low.

If the economic returns to a provider (income or profit) are invariant to the number of services he provides, little can be said about his output decisions. Consequently, it is difficult to make predictions concerning the probable utilization pattern under the arrangements in row B other than to say that more services are likely to be demanded and delivered under systems in BB than under those in BA. An example of BA or BB would be the outpatient department of a hospital being paid on a full cost reimbursement formula. (This is the pattern, for example, in New York City hospitals.) In that setting, the remuneration of medical personnel is not normally a function of the number of services they produce. Their decisions concerning utilization are therefore not subject to any financial incentives. Pauly[11] has suggested that under such an arrangement, the individual physician would have an incentive to minimize the amount of labor, or disutility-generating procedures he performs. That is, in fact, an argument that is sometimes advanced in opposition to socialized health services (such as those in England or the Soviet Union) in general, and to salaried medical practice in particular. The author's view is that the potential merits and pitfalls of salaried medical practice in this country can be inferred from the relative merits and demerits of salaried pedagogy. The typical academic department in a university is really nothing other than a multispecialty, pedagogic group practice whose members are paid a salary. University professors are likely to give that system a clean bill of health, and society seems indeed to have been served reasonably well by its pedagogues. It has to be conceded, however, that some clients of the system (namely students), often do complain that individual providers (professors) tend to shy away from disutility generating labor: the proper teaching of undergraduates and the careful reading of papers and examinations. Eliot Freidson[12] has argued eloquently that (salaried) physicians in group medical practices may become similarly insensitive to their patients' real needs.

Under arrangements CB and AA the consumers' and providers' incentives work in the same direction. Under CB, providers are likely to prescribe and consumers are likely to demand a relatively large number of services per episode of illness or per capita. Unless physical constraints to utilization are imposed by limiting supply (e.g., by holding the physician–population ratio to a given level, or by limiting the supply of hospital beds) or by still different mechanisms (such as the recently instituted PSROs), any health care program administered under financial arrangement CB is thus likely to result in high per capita resource costs. It is probable that the newly incepted provincial health programs in Canada—typically incorporating financial arrangement CB—will eventually run into difficulties because of this upward pressure on costs.

Finally, under system AA both providers and consumers face incentives to minimize the utilization of services per episode of illness or per capita. In a prepaid plan that levies a significant utilization fee on subscribers—a fee large enough to influence consumers and yet small enough not to move providers out of cell AA—one would therefore expect to find relatively low treatment costs per episode of illness or per capita.

Financial Incentives and Efficiency in the Production of Health Care

The preceding generalizations were predicated on the assumption that the provider's choice of a production technology is not influenced by the manner in which he is paid for his services. This assumption will now be relaxed, since the method of paying for medical services usually does influence the relative efficiency with which whatever services are demanded are being produced.

Standard economic theory suggests that any profit-oriented producer who sells his output in return for a predetermined price—set by third-party payers or by competitive markets—or who faces at least some market constraint in his price setting (for example, a monopolist) will produce whatever output he does produce in as efficient a manner as possible. The reasoning is that whatever revenue the output will fetch, the producer cannot but gain by producing it as cheaply as possible.

By contrast, it is reasonable to suppose that any producer who is paid for his output on a full cost reimbursement formula (row C) will show no great concern over the efficiency (or lack of it) with which his output is produced. Since hospitals are typically so reimbursed, it is often suggested that that sector would remain inefficient even if the professionalization of hospital personnel no longer imposed institutional barriers to an efficient use of health personnel. The fact that the average cost of an outpatient visit at New York City hospitals exceeded $30 in 1970 and was as high as $60 in some hospitals also probably reflects the full-cost reimbursement formulas enjoyed by these providers. Finally, one would suppose that private medical practitioners who can raise their fees with impunity (and can hence pass on to consumers any added costs due to inefficiency) are likely to organize their practice not with a view towards economy in the use of resources (including their own time), but so as to suit their own taste in these matters. Depending on the manner in which fee-for-service reimbursement by third-party payers on the basis of "customary local fees" is administered, such a system can easily approximate a mere "cost-pass-through" system.

But even in cases where providers are not reimbursed on an automatic full-cost basis or cannot push prices up at will, a penchant for efficiency cannot be assumed. In the frictionless world of economic theory the discovery and maintenance of efficiency is usually thought to be costless: It merely amounts to choosing from known alternatives the least-cost combination of medical resources (inputs) capable of producing given rates of output (services). In the real world, however, the search for efficiency is usually not costless; it requires a special effort and often generates friction within one's organization. In private medical practices, furthermore, the administration of what would objectively be deemed an optimally sized paramedical staff may be viewed by the physician as a headache of sorts, and the physician may well be inclined to trade off some income for the sake of a more tranquil practice, particularly if some or all of the resulting cost increase can be shared with consumers or taxpayers.

The gist of the preceding remarks is that the relative degree of efficiency found among providers in rows A and C is likely to vary directly with the relative degree of economic pressure on these providers. One might suppose that a provider who renders his services on a prepaid capitation basis (row C in Table 1) would not only urge his patients to exercise economy in the use of medical services, but also exercise the utmost economy himself in the production of whatever services patients do receive, and generally be more efficient than providers under systems in row A. It turns out, however, that this intuitively appealing hypothesis finds little support in the empirical record of well-known, prepaid, group practice plans. The organization of health care production in these plans and the average cost of individual services are not found to differ substantially from those in private fee-for-service practice.[13] Conceivably, the economic pressure on these plans has never been sufficiently strong to overcome an organization's inherent penchant for internal inefficiency (as distinct from the less painful efficiency in the use of services by patients). Indeed, one could conceive of a situation in which fee-for-service providers face sufficiently low predetermined fees to induce in them greater productive efficiency than might be observed for prepaid plans who are somehow financially well off, either because they enjoy a market monopoly or because they are subsidized out of public funds. It is a possibility that should generate some anxiety among those who would seek to demonstrate the economic superiority of HMOs through a massive infusion of public funds in support of that type of delivery system.

A Timid Prognosis

One major thrust of recent reform proposals for the U.S. health system has been to move the ambulatory care segment of that system from predominance of fee-for-service reimbursement towards predominance of prepayment for comprehensive health care, that is, from cell CA in Table 1 to cell AB. Both the current U.S. administration and leading spokesmen for the opposition have identified themselves with this proposal. Authoritative students of the health care sector have lent their support to the proposal as well.

Prepayment for comprehensive health care is thought to have the positive effect of forcing providers to take as their goal the maintenance of their patients' health, rather than the delivery of some narrow spectrum of services. The proposal is based on the recognition that a clear distinction must be drawn between efficiency in the production of health services and efficiency in the production of health, and that it is not enough merely to confront health care providers with incentives to produce specific services efficiently; that arrangement might still permit the delivery of an inefficient overall combination of health services. The great advantage claimed for prepayment plans such as the Kaiser Foundation Plan or the Health Insurance Plan of Greater New York (HIP) is that the financial incentives faced by these providers forces them to optimize over the entire range of medical services normally produced by a health care system. The positive effect this optimization process appears to have on the mix of ambulatory and inpatient care has been documented in numerous studies.[10] There is also some speculation that this arrangement will lead, over the longer run, to a desirable trade-off between preventive and therapeutic care. This rather powerful incentive toward global efficiency in health maintenance is probably the single most important factor rendering prepaid comprehensive group practice so attractive to many health experts.

One's enthusiasm for this obviously attractive financial arrangement, however, is tempered somewhat by two considerations. First, it was already noted above that the prepaid plans now in existence have been surprisingly unimaginative in reducing the cost of producing health services. Reasons for their failure to respond to the financial incentives they face in theory merit careful analysis in future research. Second, it is clear that a cost-conscious provider under prepayment may unduly discourage the utilization of health services, possibly at the expense of the consumer's health. All available evidence on existing prepaid, group practice plans suggests that the strong incentive to minimize costs in that setting has not so far resulted in an observable decline in the quality of care.[14] But it is well to keep in mind that many physicians now practicing in prepaid plans do so in order to prove a point: that prepaid group practice is a superior mode of medical practice. As Herbert Klarman[15] has observed on one occasion:

> To the extent . . . that physicians who have been attracted to the prepaid group practice do *differ* from other physicians . . . a sizable expansion in prepaid group practice which would draw on the other physicians might fail to yield the expected [effects].

Whether the HMO concept will in fact become the predominant delivery system in this country is another matter entirely, the obvious appeal of that concept notwithstanding. If this author had to predict the financial arrangement likely to predominate under whatever national health insurance scheme this nation will adopt, he would place his bet on system CB in Table 1. Under that system consumers will face zero or negligible out-of-pocket costs each time they consume medical services, while the bulk of non-institutional providers—and certainly the bulk of medical practitioners—will be reimbursed on a fee-for-service basis. This system seems most conformable with political realities in the United States.

Among voters and consumers a system of this sort has enormous political appeal. It generates the illusion that there is such a thing as a free lunch, and many consumers will indeed enjoy what they perceive as free nibbles. At the same time, the system also preserves at least some superficial trappings of the rugged individualism of which the medical profession prides itself: The system permits the individual physician a fair amount of control over his take from the collective health fund. Even if in the immediate future a national health insurance scheme in this country were to impose high coinsurance rates or deductibles upon consumers, such cost sharing would undoubtedly erode under continued political pressure. In the end, the financial arrangement for health care in this country is thus likely to finish at precisely the point the Canadian provinces boldly adopted as their starting point. Of all conceivable financial arrangements, it is the one least likely to induce efficiency in the production of health services or to encourage economy in their use.

FEE-FOR-SERVICE REIMBURSEMENT UNDER NATIONAL HEALTH INSURANCE

In view of the prognosis tendered above, some further comments on fee-for-service reimbursement are probably in order. These comments will be pertinent also to existing federal health programs, such as Medicaid or Part B of Medicare. To keep matters simple, it is assumed that all residents are covered by federally administered, comprehensive health insurance under which non-institutional providers of health services are reimbursed on a fee-for-service basis and consumers face zero deductibles and coinsurance rates. The latter assumption enables one to focus solely on providers. Since the latter are predominantly physicians, the terms "non-institutional providers" and "physicians" will be used interchangeably.

Under the scenario envisaged here, those in charge of administering the fee-for-service system face both enormous problems and unique opportunities. The problems lie primarily in the development of a sensible fee schedule. The opportunities lie in the financial incentives that schedule inevitably incorporates. The schedule can obviously be used to influence the organization of health care delivery in this country, and that is no trivial policy lever.

In exploring these problems and opportunities further, it is useful to proceed in terms of the two main features of any fee schedule: (1) the absolute fee level incorporated into that schedule, and (2) the structure of relative fees underlying the schedule. It is furthermore helpful in the ensuing discussion to distinguish between two administratively distinct types of fee schedules:

A. a fixed schedule of fees negotiated between some third-party payer (presumably the federal government or its agents) and representatives of the non-institutional providers of health care, uniformly applied to all providers, or deliberately differentiated by specific localities and/or medical specialties; and

B. the set of fee schedules emerging under an administratively loose system, such as reimbursement of individual providers on the basis of "reasonable customary local fees." Such schedules are not negotiated; they are tolerated.

Schedules of type A are thought to cover all medical specialties. Schedules of type B may, of course, be averaged and I shall occasionally refer to that average as "the fee schedule."

The Overall Absolute Level of the Fee Schedule

Given the number of non-institutional providers (physicians) and given the number and mix of services they produce, the overall absolute fee level stakes out the claim physicians as a group are granted on the goods and services available to society as a whole. Under the insurance scheme envisaged here, the financial resources so transferred flow through the public sector and will hence appear as a cost item in some agency's budget. It is this budget item with which Congress and the media are typically concerned and to which they refer as "the cost of non-institutional care."

This so-called budget cost, which indicates the value of goods and services the nonphysician sector of society must transfer to its physician sector, is not to be confused with the real resource costs of the services rendered by non-institutional providers. The latter are properly measured only by the goods and services that could have been produced if the capital equipment and manpower actually used by the physician sector had never been employed there but instead had been applied to whatever would have been the next best alternative use (not necessarily medical) of these resources. They are the goods and services society as a whole gives up to have a non-institutional provider sector in the first place.

It should be obvious that, other things being equal, the real resource costs of non-institutional health care are not sensitive to the absolute fee level, nor to the budget costs that do vary directly with absolute fees. Unfortunately, "other things" do not remain constant when the absolute fee level changes. Such changes determine the average financial reward earned per physician, and that reward in turn serves actual and potential physicians as an economic signal directly influencing their behavior. In particular, the average financial reward earned per provider (physician) is (1) one of the more important determinants of the aggregate supply of providers (physicians), where *aggregate* may refer either to the nation as a whole, or to a particular locality, or to a particular medical specialty; and (2) one of many determinants that influence the average productivity of providers, defined here as the number of services produced per year. Thus, in the longer run, the setting of an absolute average fee level determines not only the distribution of that legendary pie called net national product among members of society, but also the very size and composition of that pie.

Precisely what determines the overall level of fees currently charged by American physicians is as yet an open question among economists. According to one theory, this level is determined in rough and ready fashion by market forces. An alternative theory is that the typical American physician operates under conditions of excess demand for his services, therefore has a fair amount of discretionary power over his fees, and sets the latter so as to attain some target income. The second of these theories leaves the determination of the target income unexplained. It is typically assumed that this target is set with reference to the income distribution in the physician's locality.

Whichever theory is more nearly correct, it is reasonable to assume that the uninsured patient's financial position does exert a subtle constraint on the physician's pricing policy. It has long been known that this constraint is eroded by third-party payment. Under the insurance scheme envisaged here, the overall absolute fee level negotiated under type A schedules—or that tolerated under type B schedules—will in fact be a reflection of what a handful of legislators, administrators, and representatives of the medical profession consider an "adequate physician income." Just how "adequate" will be defined in this context is an intriguing question.

From the viewpoint of the medical profession, it would seem logical to define an adequate physician income as one that preserves the physician's customary position in the nation's overall income distribution. In arguing for that definition, physicians could cite philosophers David Hume and Adam Smith who, incidentally, furnished also the further rationale that

> The long time and great expense which must be laid out in their [the physician's] education, when combined with this circumstance [the need for trust] necessarily still further enhance the price [that should be] paid for their labour.[5]

It seems reasonable to suppose that, under the insurance scheme envisaged here, the medical profession would be successful in implementing that definition. It is well known that a medical education is arduous and imposes upon the trainee substantial private costs. Much would probably be made of this fact in negotiations over fee schedules. Other professionals do, of course, also bear stiff private costs in obtaining their training. But few of these professionals have been quite as successful as physicians seem to be in persuading the public that to amortize his or her high training costs, society practically owes the graduate a secure and decent living. The reason for this lack of success is not far to seek. In pushing the argument, pedagogues may point to the wonders they create in the mind of youth and aerospace scientists to their role in the nation's security. Such arguments, however, are far too abstract and do not wash in the public's mind, certainly not in Peoria.

Physicians, on the other hand, typically play a highly personal and usually highly beneficial role in their patient's lives. One may suppose that therefore both the public and third-party payers can much more readily be persuaded to the notion that 12 years or more of arduous training merit a decent financial reward. And if one may judge by other nations already operating insurance systems such as that envisaged here—for example West Germany—then a "decent reward" will in all likelihood always be understood to mean a position somewhere near the top of the national income scale. In West Germany, for example, the average physician income is reported to be about $65,000.[16] Given the average income of West Germans, this is a high income indeed.

If arguments over the definition of an "adequate physician income" merely involved the size of the transfer payment from society to physicians, one could shrug it off as part of the massive zero-sum game played annually by unions all over the nation. Unfortunately, in the scenario painted above the negotiators may very well abstract entirely from demand and supply conditions in the health manpower area. The more generous the supply of physicians will be relative to the demand for them, the lower will of course be each physician's share in the common patient pool. Such a development would in all likelihood exert an enormous upward pressure on the profession's demand for fee increases and one need not be a complete cynic to predict that negotiated or tolerated fees would ultimately be permitted to reach a level capable of generating the desired target income. By thus robbing the income figure of its ability to signal any excess supply conditions to potential entrants into the profession, a seemingly innocent fee policy aimed merely at maintaining the status quo would therefore unwittingly ratify a continuous inflation in the real resource costs of health maintenance. It is not too farfetched to suggest that, with passive assistance from existing third-party payers (private insurance carriers, Blue Shield, and Medicare/Medicaid), this scenario has already been played out for many years in the field of general surgery.

The scenario just described should render much more attractive the economist's hard-nosed definition of adequacy, to wit: *in any medical specialty, and in any geographic region, net income per physician is adequate when it elicits a supply of physician services just sufficient to meet society's medically legitimate need for them.* On this definition the absolute fee level is not treated as a mere adjustment factor used to reconcile whatever supply of medical manpower there may be with the target income that manpower desires, but instead as a policy instrument employed to equate the supply of physician services to the demand (need) for them. The potential of using negotiated (or tolerated) fee schedules in this way is one of the opportunities alluded to in the introduction of this section.

Absolute Fee Levels and the Supply of Medical Manpower Each year a large number of perfectly qualified applicants to American medical schools are rejected for want of medical school capacity. In recent years the rejection–application ratio has risen drastically. Medical educators view this trend with alarm. It is argued that to deny qualified young Americans the opportunity to come to the aid of their suffering fellow men is a national shame and downright "inimical to our democratic institutions."[17] The suggested remedy is a further massive infusion of federal funds into the already highly subsidized medical education sector.

It is easy to be sympathetic to these educators' complaint. From their vantage point they see a seriously imbalanced market for medical educations in which demand far outstrips supply and the latter is not permitted to adjust to the former. Furthermore one has understanding for the fact that, just as aerospace engineers can never be persuaded that there is such a thing as excess armament, so the medical educator finds it hard to believe that there can really be too much of a good thing: medical manpower. And just as the aerospace engineer can buttress his case by pointing to the bellicose Russian, the inscrutable Chinese, and the fanatic Arab, so the medical educator can point to crowded waiting rooms, to unattended patients in center cities or the rural hinterland, and to the many foreign-trained physicians tending to our hospitals. Either case has much plausibility, and one may be inclined to believe Professor Alex Gerber's recent assertion that "Yes! There is a Physician Shortage."[18]

The case can be put, however, that the current alarm over a physician shortage *at the aggregate* level is much exaggerated and that, at that level, the United States currently finds itself in a position or will soon find itself in the position of a mild physician surplus.[19] It has long been recognized among careful analysts that the perceived physician shortage in this country is really evidence of a severe maldistribution of medical manpower, compounded by widespread inefficiency in the use of that manpower. And although one would not wish to make light of the compassion shown by potential entrants into the medical profession, careful analysis of the locational pattern among physicians suggests that, on balance, that compassion gravitates heavily towards patients residing in culturally or geographically attractive locations and able to pay for the physician's ministrations. One who is part of a community of teacher–scholars who lavish their considerable pedagogic talents on those least in need of it does not find the locational preferences of physicians shameful. It is merely suggested that locationally isolated health manpower shortages ought not to be cited as evidence of an overall physician shortage, or as a reason for continued medical school expansion.

If one accepts the proposition that there may not be an overall physician shortage in this country after all, one is left with the problems of imbalance in the market for medical educations and of the maldistribution of medical manpower. Here it is well to recall that a person's choice of an occupation is motivated by a good many factors, among them the individual's intrinsic interest in the occupation itself, the prestige society accords that occupation, the cost of entering the occupation, and last, but by no means least, the financial rewards it offers.

It has been estimated that the expected average annual rate of return to a qualified college graduate's investment (including foregone earnings) in four years of medical school and one year of internship is currently about 25 percent.[20] This is a handsome return by almost any standard, for it is hard to think of any other professional career offering so high a rate of return with such relative certainty. Although it would be difficult to disentangle, for any cohort of medical school applicants, their compassion for the ill from a healthy instinct for good investment opportunities, it is also difficult to suppress the thought that many an applicant's innate compassion is heightened by the prospect of high financial reward. In fact, one feels entitled to the hypothesis that the current imbalance in the market for medical educations suggests either that current medical fees are on average much too high, or that the private costs of a medical education are much too low. Either variable could be used to bring that market into a more reasonable balance.

If it were attempted to reduce the demand for medical educations by having medical students shoulder a greater share of their currently heavily subsidized training, one could use the higher tuition charges as a lever to bring about a more desirable distribution of physicians across regions or medical specialties. One way to achieve this would be to couple the increase in tuition with a generous loan program under which part or all of the loan could ultimately be forgiven in return for service in an underdoctored area or specialty.

The immediate objection to the tuition proposal is that it would send candidates from the lower or middle income classes "into the country," so to speak, leaving the culturally more attractive regions to the fortunate offspring of more opulent parents. There is something to that objection. The obvious alternative to the proposal, especially under national health insurance, would be to stratify fee schedules by region and/or specialty and to use differentials in the absolute fee level as an instrument to bring about the desired redistribution. This proposal has much potential. There is evidence that in Canada, where the introduction of national health insurance has brought about greater geographic uniformity in fee schedules, the expected redistribution of medical manpower is already under way. There is no reason to suppose that a bold application of this scheme in the United States would not be equally effective.

The current operation of this country's fee-for-service system—including the reimbursement formulas adopted by the Medicare and Medicaid programs—are almost designed to engender the much lamented maldistribution of medical facilities. As Table 2 indicates, "customary fees" tend to be relatively high in localities with relatively high physician–population ratios, and relatively low in areas with low physician density. As noted earlier, there is as yet no universally accepted explanation for this pattern. Some analysts hypothesize that fees are largely market-determined and physician density adjusts to local fees, while others argue that physician density is best explained by other locational variables and fees adjust to physican density. Precisely which way causation runs in this case is actually not crucial to the policy measure under discussion here, and that policy consists of the setting of absolute fee levels in a way that (1) brings the aggregate demand for medical educations more into balance with the nation's actual overall demand for medical manpower, and (2) provides physicians with sufficiently strong financial incentives to locate where physicians are needed and to practice in a specialty whose services are needed.

TABLE 2 Regional Differences in Physician Density, Fees, and Practice Patterns

		Census Division		
	Year	New England	East–North Central	East–South Central
No. active M.D.'s involved in patient care (per 100,000 population)	1970	161	115	95
Average fee for a routine follow-up visit ($)				
General practice		6.79	6.29	5.21
Internal medicine		9.40	8.05	7.20
Pediatrics		7.53	6.94	5.40
General surgery		9.76	7.76	6.85
Obstetrics/gynecology		9.77	9.32	7.60
Average No. aides per physician	1967	1.3	1.8	2.1
Annual No. patient visits per M.D.				
Total visits	1969	4,808	6,611	8,408
Office visits		384	4,799	6,052

SOURCE: Reinhardt UE: Physician Productivity and the "Physician Shortage" (forthcoming from Ballinger Publishing Company), Table 2-5, Chapter II.

Absolute Fee Levels and Physician Productivity One factor that complicates the already difficult policy task described above is the fact that absolute fee levels can influence both the overall supply and distribution of physicians and the economic behavior of the individual physician. The conventional textbook model of the profit-maximizing firm suggests that the firm's (provider's) rate of output increases in response to increases in the price of his output, or at least that it will not fall. Those who remember this model may therefore fear that any attempt to lower the overall absolute level of medical fees would have the unintended side effect of lowering the annual average output of services per physician. Fortunately or unfortuantely, matters are not quite that straightforward in the case of medical practice. Two factors in particular render predictions for that type of "business firm" hazardous:

1. the typical medical practice is owner-operated; and
2. as noted in section II, the practice setup preferred by the physician (particularly the extent of task delegation to auxiliary personnel) may deviate from what an objective observer would deem the economically most efficient mode. If the absolute fee level is such as to afford the physician a satisfactory income without complete efficiency, he may well decide to forego further financial gains from greater efficiency for the sake of a more congenial practice setup.

Even if one abstracts completely from factor 2, the theory of owner-operated enterprises suggests that the owner's time input (physician hours per year) and his rate of output may either increase, remain unchanged, or decrease in response to a given change in the price of his output (i.e., absolute fees). Economists depict this phenomenon by a so-called backward-bending supply-of-hours curve, such as that in Figure 1. In that diagram it is assumed that up to fee level F_1, increases in fees will elicit added work effort from the physician. Increases in fees beyond F_1, on the other hand, are thought to decrease his work effort. The odd shape of the curve is thought to result from a continuous struggle of the so-called "income effect" with the so-called "substitution effect." Other things being equal, a fee increase raises the physician's income, which in turn may induce him to enjoy some extra leisure without depressing income below its previous level. This is the "income effect" of a fee change. A fee increase, however, also increases the rate at which leisure can be converted into income (hourly remuneration) which is an incentive for added work effort. This is the "substitution effect." Up to F_1, the substitution effect is thought to

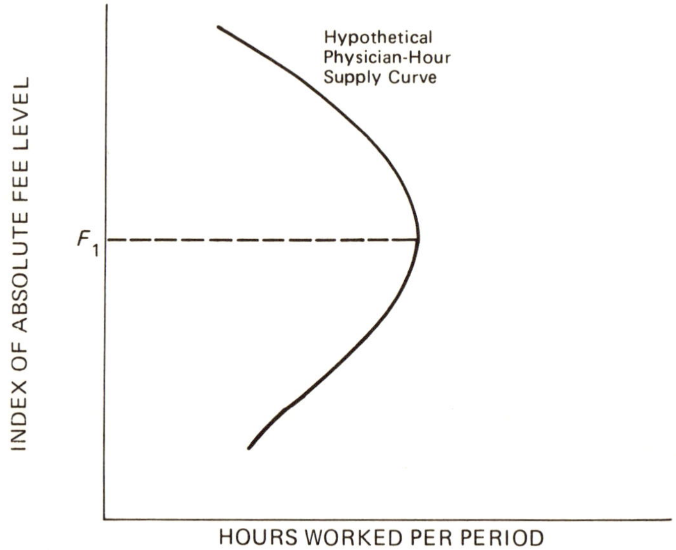

FIGURE 1 Supply-of-hours curve.

overcome the income effect. Thereafter, the income effect is thought to dominate.

Without knowing the exact shape of the physician's labor supply curve, it is impossible to predict the effect any given change in the absolute fee level will have on his work effort. Empirical research on this issue has not so far revealed conclusively whether American physicians are, on balance, situated on the upward-sloping or the backward-bending segment of their labor supply curve. It is anybody's guess what work response a lowering of the overall absolute fee level would elicit from the typical American physician.

Figure 1 depicts only the hypothetical response of physician hours to changes in absolute fees. To translate this response into medical services produced is rather difficult, for the extent of task delegation (and hence the physician's hourly productivity) must be assumed to vary in response to both changes in his hours and changes in the absolute fee level. Formal economic models of physician behavior suggest that, other things (including the fee level) being equal, an increase in physician hours per period should increase the marginal contribution auxiliary personnel can make to a physician's practice, so that he should be inclined to employ correspondingly more auxiliary personnel time.[21] The same theory also suggests that, other things (including physician hours) being equal, an increase in the absolute level of fees should enable the physician to afford more auxiliary personnel. If both hours and the fee level move in the same direction, the amount of auxiliary personnel time used should move in the same direction as well, and so should the physician's annual output of services. On the other hand, if hours and fees move in opposite directions—as they would on the backward-bending part of the physician-hour supply curve—there are two opposing effects on the employment of auxiliary personnel. No unambiguous prediction can be made concerning either the net effect on employment or the physician's annual rate of output (unless, of course, one had a completely specified and estimated model of the physician's behavior—a pipe dream at this time.)

The gist of the preceding paragraphs is that the effect of changes in absolute fee levels on physician productivity cannot be predicted unambiguously. The model on which that conclusion is based, however, is rather stylized and may evoke no little bemusement in this audience. It is this author's view, based in part on his own research and also on that of other analysts,[22] that the typical physician in this country has not pushed task delegation to the extent that seems both medically sound and economically justifiable (see factor 2 above). One probable reason for this failure to economize is that there has never been sufficient economic pressure on individual providers to economize, a theme already developed.

An alert and objective observer can hardly fail to perceive the enormous opportunity the administration of a type A fee schedule would offer in this area. It is not too difficult to incorporate a penchant for internal inefficiency formally into the behavioral model sketched out above,[23] and a model so enriched suggests that the supply curve for physician services is likely to be backward-bending for a much longer stretch than the earlier version of the model suggests. In concrete terms, this means that there is the distinct possibility that ceilings on absolute fees could be used as a policy instrument, literally leaving a physician bent on maintaining or improving his income no alternative other than to enhance the productivity of his practice—presumably through more effective use of paramedical personnel or through whatever other means seem suitable.

The policy described (and not necessarily proposed) in the preceding paragraph may strike the reader as hideous, and tough it undoubtedly is. Even so, objectivity forces the analyst to bring it to the attention of this audience. Furthermore, the objective observer will discover in this policy nothing other than the idea to simulate exactly the kind of economic pressure to which truly competitive enterprises are exposed as a matter of course and which forces them into the high degree of efficiency commonly associated with competitive markets. This pressure is the motive force of the much praised free-enterprise system, and it is precisely this pressure that generates the alleged benificence of the Invisible Hand.

Some caveats must, however, be raised in connection with the policies described so far. Any strictly enforced ceiling on the absolute level of physician fees runs the risk of triggering either excess utilization of services or a diminution in the quality of services rendered. In the provision of medical services, it is not always easy to distinguish genuine productivity gains from increases in, say, weekly patient visits purchased at the cost of lower quality. Suppose a physician operating under conditions of excess demand were constrained by an effective fee ceiling. His response to that constraint might be either to increase the efficiency with which his practice renders services of a given intrinsic quality, or simply to be less thorough and thus to welch on that quality. (By diminution of quality I am not referring here to a reduction in the amount of physician time spent per patient visit; such a reduction is implicit in the very notion of task delegation and need in no way reduce the quality of a physician's care. I am referring instead to any undue quickening of the pace of the practice without the benefit of added task delegation. And even the latter could, of course, be pushed beyond the medically safe.)

As noted earlier, conditions of excess supply generate the additional problem of upward pressure on the per capita utilization of physician services. That pressure may remain mild to moderate if fees are permitted to rise sufficiently to afford even underemployed physicians a decent living, as seems to be the case in general surgery in at least some parts of the country.[24] To superimpose fee ceilings onto this context would clearly be to invite much more pronounced upward pressure on per capita utilization, with potentially serious consequences.

These potential side effects of fee ceilings must be explicitly taken into account in attempts to use absolute fee levels to generate a more appropriate distribution of physicians geographically or across specialties, or to induce greater efficiency in the production of ambulatory care. One suspects therefore that, were such policies implemented, they would inevitably be accompanied by some external monitoring of per capita utilization and of the quality of non-institutional health care.

The Relative Fee Structure in the Fee Schedule

It will be recalled that the fee schedule under discussion here is one thought to cover all medical services and all medical specialties. The relative fee structure underlying this schedule should obey the following principles:

1. Services that are identical in terms of objectively determined standards of quality and in terms of their medical content should be covered by one and only one fee, regardless of how they are produced.
2. There should be strict proportionality between the fees for medical services and their resource costs.
3. The definition and measurement of resource costs (primarily the time of physicians and paramedical personnel, and supplies, including an allowance for the amortization of fixed costs) should be based on an objectively efficient mode of production.

A fourth principle, namely that the profit margin implicit in the fee schedule be such as to equate the supply of medical services with the demand for them has already been discussed under the rubric of "absolute fee levels."

One Fee for One Type of Service At a glance the logic of the first principle seems too self-evident to warrant further elaboration. A loaf of bread should have a given price regardless of whether it was baked by a master baker, a journeyman, or an apprentice. Such particulars of the production process are not a relevant dimension from the consumer's viewpoint.

In the context of health care production, on the other hand, the production process itself is widely viewed as an important dimension of product–quality as perceived by the patient. Thus it is thought that a routine appendectomy, if performed by a general surgeon, is a service quite distinct from one performed by a general practitioner and hence warrants a differential in remuneration. Similarly, it is thought that the suturing of a simple cut by a physician is a service quite distinct from the suturing of that same cut by a fully qualified physician assistant, and therefore also warrants a differential in fees. The intrinsic difference, one supposes, is thought to lie in the quality of the services.

The crucial question here is whose conception of quality is most relevant. It is conceivable that a careful medical audit reveals no difference in the intrinsic quality of the services described above. It can rightfully be held, therefore, that the appendectomies should be reimbursed at the same rate, regardless of who performed them, and similarly for the suturing. There should be a differential only if the expected (actuarial) quality of the general surgeon's operation is thought to differ from the general practitioner's.

The patient's perception in these matters may unfortunately deviate from that of a medical auditor. Patients may simply proceed on the premise that a specialist's care is always superior to that rendered by a generalist, regardless of the medical condition being treated. The general surgeon's appendectomy would therefore be more highly ranked on the quality scale, and this ranking could be used as the basis for a fee differential.

Economists customarily view the consumer's psyche as the ultimate determinant of the value of goods or services. An economist's natural inclination may therefore be to graft this valuation principle also onto medical fee schedules. The problem is that in this instance the consumer's perception tends to be highly blurred and also highly malleable. He or she is generally open to instruction on medical matters and may, in fact, view the elements of the fee schedule as a guide to evaluating the quality of particular services. For that reason it would seem more appropriate to entrust the definition of quality care to the competent medical auditor, and to structure the fee schedule on the latter's perception. The principle ought to apply not only to the differentiation of fees by medical specialty, but also to the setting of fees for services performed by an assistant under a physician's supervision, as long as the physician is held legally responsible for the quality of these services.

In connection with physician assistants, one would be remiss in failing to comment here on the government's pricing policy for services rendered under Part B of the Medicare program. It appears that, according to the Social Security Administration's (SSA's) original interpretation of Title XVIII of the Medicare Act, the suturing of a simple wound, if performed by a physician, is something quite distinct indeed from the suturing of that same wound by a qualified physician assistant: Under the SSA's interpretation, the former service warrants full reimbursement at the physician's regular fee, while the latter does not warrant any payment at all.[25]

It is not easy even after searching rumination to infer a plausible motive for this peculiar pricing policy. A facetious explanation would be to ascribe the policy to that "sinister force" allegedly on the loose in the nation's capital. Conceivably that force is bent on destroying any possibility of inducing greater efficiency into the production of the nation's ambulatory care. For, let there be no mistake about it, a policy of reimbursing non-institutional providers of care at "reasonable customary local fees" (with the word "reasonable" quite generously interpreted), combined with a refusal to pay for the performance of properly delegated tasks is not likely to fail in reaching that sinister objective.

It would be helpful if the intention behind the SSA interpretation were indeed wicked, for one calls to mind here sociologist Marion Levy's[26] famous *Fourth Law of the Disillusionment of the True Liberal:*

> ALWAYS PRAY THAT YOUR OPPOSITION BE WICKED.
> IN WICKEDNESS THERE IS A STRONG
> STRAIN TOWARD RATIONALITY.
> THEREFORE THERE IS ALWAYS THE
> POSSIBILITY, IN THEORY, OF HANDLING
> THE WICKED BY OUTTHINKING THEM.

Unfortunately the SSA intention seems to have been anything but wicked. One suspects that its interpretation of Title XVIII was intended to save the taxpayer money.[27] Here it must be recalled that legislators and administrators think primarily in terms of budget costs and that their position usually forces them to work within short time horizons. The reasoning in this instance appears to have been that to reimburse the physician his regular fee for a service that is wholly performed by a physician assistant would merely serve to inflate the cost of ambulatory care and, besides, bestow upon the physician an undeserved windfall profit.

If one thinks of the very, very short run in which the supply of physician assistants is given, and if one further assumes that physicians already employing such assistants will retain them come what may, then the SSA pricing policy in this respect would indeed be helpful to the taxpayer (in that very same short run). Taxpayers would receive something (namely, ambulatory care produced by physician assistants) for nothing, and that would clearly be to the good.

Unfortunately, the SSA pricing policy has long-run implications that run directly counter to the government's policy of subsidizing the training of physician assistants and of encouraging their employment. It is obvious that failure to reimburse physicians for tasks properly delegated to qualified assistants substantially reduces the economic potential of such assistants from the individual physician's perspective. It may therefore be expected that physician assistants, upon completion of their highly subsidized training, will find only a lukewarm reception among potential employers. Given the resistance among patients and physicians to the physician assistant on still other grounds, the SSA pricing policy therefore confronts this manpower with yet another unnecessary hurdle.

If it were true that the "windfall profit" earned by the physician under full-fee reimbursement would, through the income effect already discussed earlier, induce the physician to convert all of the productivity gains from task delegation into added leisure, then the entire physician assistant program would of course come to naught one way or another. There would be no net increase in output per physician and fees would not fall. That result, however, surely represents an extreme. The more probable outcome would be a mere partial conversion of productivity gains into added physician leisure, and sizeable additions to the supply of ambulatory health services without increases in fees. Physicians employing physician assistants would obviously reap some additional income from that employment, but the hardnosed economist would view that result as perfectly appropriate. The extra income, after all, would reward relatively greater efficiency. It would, in fact, pay the physician for his assistance in reducing the long-run real resource costs of ambulatory care in this country, for in the long-run the substitution of paramedical for medical manpower is apt to reduce the real resource cost of health care production. In other words, an economist is inclined to view the pricing policy (that is, principle 1 above), rejected by SSA as unfair and inflationary, as eminently fair and, in the long run, probably deflationary.

Before leaving this topic it must be mentioned that, subsequent to the original SSA ruling, legislation was passed instructing the Department of Health, Education, and Welfare to experiment with alternative reimbursement modes for physician assistants. The intent of that legislation seems to be to discover some partial reimbursement rate sufficient not to discourage the acceptance of the physician assistant concept among physicians, and yet below the rate paid the physician for the performance of the identical service. Such partial reimbursement would obviously be an improvement over the present policy, in the sense that to sin only three times a week seems better than to sin daily.

As a first and basic principle, however, it would seem to at least this economist that one ought not to tinker thusly with the fee schedule in the hope of reducing the cost of ambulatory care. Artificial fee differentials of this sort merely serve to reinforce in the patient's mind the notion that task delegation in medical practice inevitably impairs the quality of medical care. Conveyance of this message is surely not the intent behind HEW's considerable effort in the health manpower area. If fee schedules are to be used to reduce the budget cost and the real resource cost of ambulatory care in this country, other policies suggest themselves, such as those described in the previous section. Until these more powerful policies are attempted, however, it is best to reward economic efficiency wherever it may be found generously, even if that means toleration of "windfall profits" reaped by the efficient physician.

Relative Fees and the Cost of Medical Services

The second and third principles mentioned earlier suggest that, in the construction of a fee schedule, the relative value points assigned to individual services should conform as closely as possible to the relative cost of these services. Furthermore they suggest that these unit costs should not be just an average over some sample of physicians, but instead be standards inferred from the most efficient way of producing each service. Both propositions require a few added comments.

The proposition that the relative value scales be tied closely to relative costs is motivated by the notion that, in the absence of proportionality between fees and costs, providers may bias the mix of services they prescribe toward relatively more profitable procedures. It is sometimes suggested that, relative to the time and materials costs of performing each service, the fee schedules used in the United States and Canada tend to place greater rewards on procedural items—such as surgery, injections, x rays, and laboratory tests—than on less clearly defined diagnostic services and on preventive care. In the Canadian province of Saskatchewan, for example, the average hourly remuneration for surgical work is reported to be three times as high as that for the routine work performed by general practitioners—a differential that seems out of proportion to any differences in the cost of medical training.

It may be assumed that, as long as physicians operate under conditions of excess demand and can earn a comfortable living by performing only medically necessary procedures, their practice style will remain impervious to such distortions in relative fees. On the other hand, problems may arise under conditions of excess supply, or where effective fee ceilings exert strong economic pressure on individual providers. As noted earlier, in composing the treatments for given medical conditions, physicians have considerable leeway on purely medical grounds. It may therefore be supposed that even without overtly compromising his professional ethics, the physician may in a subtle way become sensitive to the relative marginal rewards to him of medically sound alternative treatments, especially if his patients enjoy first-dollar insurance coverage and are hence indifferent to the cost of alternative treatments.

Undue differentials in the hourly remuneration implicit in fee schedules may, of course, elicit more overtly abusive practices among ethically marginal practitioners. Such differentials, for example, have long been thought to furnish the economic basis for fee-splitting between specialists and the referring generalist, and they are said to induce some general practitioners to perform surgery for which they are not trained. As a layman in medical matters this author is loath to offer any strong assertions on this point, but it may be pertinent here to quote from an address to physicians by a former president of the Canadian Medical Association:[28]

> As long as [general] practitioners are forced to resort to surgical procedures to make the difference between a bare living and a decent income, just so long will the scales be weighted against any patient who presents himself for examination. This is a failing common to all of us and one which each of us here has experienced.

Coming as it does from the president of a medical association, this statement gives one pause.

There remains the question of how the standard relative unit costs of individual medical services ought to be calculated. This is quite obviously a highly complex task and only a few superficial comments can be offered on it here.

Aside from the usual problem of allocating fixed costs to individual units of output—a problem that neither economists nor accountants have ever solved satisfactorily and which they have fudged through the ages—the main difficulty is likely to be the costing of human labor. The cost of paramedical personnel is objectively given and may be distributed over services in accordance with paramedical-aide time spent on them. It is probably not insurmountably difficult either to discover, through task analysis, the content of physician time in each efficiently produced service. The problem lies in converting these time units into costs, for the cost of physician time is not objectively given.

One approach might be to value the time of all physicians equally, regardless of medical specialty. General practitioners might rate this procedure as "equitable," but one wonders whether specialists would concur. The latter, after all, undergo more lengthy training and, in the case of surgery at least, may not be able to work as many hours per week or as many years in their life as can general practitioners, internists, or pediatricians. True equality therefore requires that one adjust for these factors.

One baseline rule that suggests itself for this purpose would be to set relative hourly remuneration for the various specialties so that, after adjustment for differentials in training costs and in tolerable workloads, the net present (discountable) value of their medical career is the same for all physicians upon completion of their internship. Under this rule, the relative hourly remuneration of any two specialties becomes a rather complex mathematical expression (available from the author) and need certainly not equal unity.

The preceding rule may, unfortunately, violate the requirement that the supply of physician services be equated to the demand for them in all medical specialties. Physicians may associate certain psychic costs and/or benefits with working in a particular specialty. To attain equilibrium in the services market, one may therefore have to allow differentials even in the net present values defined above. The required adjustments are easily made in principle, but hard to estimate in practice. A further consideration of these problems would clearly exceed the scope of this paper. At this point one can but sketch the bare outline of a standard costing procedure for medical services and note its essential features.

Throughout this section it has been assumed that the standard unit costs of a service are those inferred from an efficient production process. Concretely this means that services safely delegatable to a physician assistant should be priced as if a physician assistant actually produced it in all cases. Physicians who actually had the service produced by an assistant would fare well under this rule. On the other hand, physicians who failed to delegate tasks efficiently would obviously be penalized. In the example under consideration, if the physician produced the perfectly delegatable task himself, he would effectively sell his own time at the price of a physician assistant's time. The implicit loss might soon become obvious to him. One suspects that a fee schedule so constructed would do much to encourage a more efficient utilization of health manpower in the production of ambulatory care.

CONCLUDING REMARKS

The impression may have been gained by now that behind this paper's arid prose there lurks the mind of a misanthrope, archtypical of that dismal science called economics, and out to get the medical profession. The author would prefer not to be so labeled. The fact is that he has a healthy respect for American medicine and regards the typical American physician at least as socially responsive and responsible as is the typical social scientist.

It must be remembered that the scenarios explored in the previous section were developed against the assumed backdrop of comprehensive national health insurance. There is little doubt that sooner or later this nation will move toward some such insurance scheme. It may also be supposed that the transfer of financial resources from consumers to health care providers under such a system will either flow through the public sector or will at least be monitored by it. There will be perennial arguments over the appropriate absolute size of this transfer and over its distribution among providers.

It is inconceivable that the public sector will choose to act under these circumstances simply as a transfer agent, leaving to the health care providers the determination of the absolute size of the transfer and of its distribution among them. To do so would literally be giving health care providers collectively and individually a key to the public treasury. It should not be supposed that under these circumstances hospital administrators and physicians would comport themselves any less responsibly than would any other group of professionals or, for that matter, any other citizen granted unfettered access to the public purse. The problem is that health care providers would probably not act more responsibly than their fellowmen either, and therein lies the danger.

It is clear that if every provider in some group of providers wished to earn at least as much as the group's average income—and that does not strike one as an immodest or socially irresponsible posture—then that average would drift inexorably up over time. Among any group of professionals, however, there are those whose income expectations far exceed the average and, indeed, any reasonable bounds. Unfortunately their characteristics—and their income—become part of the relevant average and as such exert an upward pull on it. It would be reassuring, for example, if at least occasionally one read that one of those radiologists or pathologists reportedly carrying home incomes in the hundreds of thousands do what they ought to do: blush (or if responsible spokesmen of the medical profession commented critically on such incomes). Alas, one does not come across such stories and hence one worries that today's outrage may easily become tomorrow's norm, almost regardless of the social ethics of individual health care providers.

It is patently obvious that today's citizenry and its legislative representatives share these worries, and that any national health insurance scheme will in fact be accompanied by fairly strict control over budget costs. The attempt in the last section has been to present a broad sketch of the various forms such cost monitoring can take. It is obvious that under a regular fee-for-service system these controls can be formidable and pervasive.

I have always found the medical profession's support of the fee-for-service system puzzling. Not only does professional support of that system—particularly the assertion that it is the *sine qua non* of high-quality care—lend itself to a variety of interpretations, some of which are quite unflattering, but the system also furnishes the most convenient vehicle anyone could wish for lay control over the medical profession. For it should be obvious that under comprehensive health insurance with fee-for-service reimbursement, details of every physician–patient contact will be recorded in some computerized data bank. There is no need to elaborate upon the many possibilities such a data bank furnishes.

The alternatives to fee-for-service reimbursement are prepayment and/or salaried medical practice. The author has to concede that, after the preceding survey, these payment modes do hold a certain attraction, their own inherent dangers notwithstanding. Under a fee-for-service system, revenue (income) equals price (fee) times quantity (services), and cost-conscious administrators will ultimately wish to regulate individual providers with respect to both price and quantity. Under prepayment or salaried practice, cost control as such does not require a monitoring of quantity at all. The latter would be necessary only if it were suspected that health care providers underprescribe or otherwise welsh on quality.

A system somewhere in between is one now operating in West Germany. Under that system a great many insurance companies and "sickness funds" (Krankenkassen) collect premiums from consumers, but pool these at the state (Land) level and turn them over to the state's medical association (Land Aerztekammern) for distribution among its members on a fee-for-service basis. The size of the overall transfer is negotiated annually between associations of the insurance carriers and the medical associations, and requires implicit or explicit government approval. The absolute fee level is determined as the quotient of the available fund divided by services delivered. From the insurer's (administrator's) viewpoint, this system is akin to a salary or a prepayment system. From the physician's viewpoint, it is a fee-for-service system, but one with a peculiar twist: The system effectively places the entire profession into a massive annual zero-sum game. Since one physician's gain is another's loss, individual physicians naturally are subjected to rather strict peer review. This peer review focuses exclusively on quantity of services delivered.

It may be suggested that the West German system is really an HMO of the American medical foundation variety. That is almost correct. The difference between our notion of a medical foundation and the West German system is that the former is thought to operate in a competitive market—or so one is told—while no pretense at competition is made under the German system. The government therefore actively controls the overall size of the financial transfer (although, as was noted earlier, not to the physician's serious disadvantage). I have argued elsewhere that if local medical foundations are implemented in this country with the assumption, wish, or prayer that there be competition in local markets and that there be no need for external cost control, then we are likely to be in for some sad surprises. A network of autonomous local medical foundations is not likely to solve the problem of maldistribution of medical services either. I would be glad to elaborate upon these propositions, but to do so here would make this yet another paper.

REFERENCES AND NOTES

1. This section draws very heavily and sometimes quotes from Reinhardt UE: Proposed changes in the organization of health care delivery, an overview and critique. Milbank Mem Fund Q 51(2):169–222, 1973.
2. Systems in which consumers bear a fixed annual deductible but no coinsurance rate cover both columns A and B.
3. If the annual capitation fee can be raised at will in the light of recent or anticipated cost experience, prepayment may take on the nature of full cost reimbursement and the entire system may shift to row B.
4. The classification of systems described here is not exhaustive. There are a number of arrangements that fall somewhere in between the limiting types shown in the table. For example, there exist remuneration schemes under which the provider's income or profit does not vary directly with each unit of service delivered, but does vary indirectly as a function of the average volume of services (or their quality) he has rendered in the past. Such providers would fall somewhere between rows B and C. Similarly, consumers may find their health insurance premiums to be a function of their past utilization of health services. For such consumers the out-of-pocket cost of health services may not vary directly with the number of services they consume, but still be determined indirectly by a lagged function of overall utilization rates. These consumers would therefore fall somewhere between columns A and B.
5. Smith A: The Wealth of Nations. New York, Random House, 1937, p 105.
6. *Ibid.*, and in Glaser WA: Paying the Doctor: Systems of Remuneration and Their Effects. Baltimore, The Johns Hopkins Press, 1970.
7. In Pauly's model, the factor most likely to lead to some erosion in the physician's ethical standards is an increase in the physician–population ratio in the physician's locality. In the absence of real excess demand, such an increase forces a larger physician pool to share a given patient pool and hence exerts downward pressure on the individual physician's patient load. Unless fees can be raised to maintain income at its customary level, there is thought to be a penchant for overprescription of services.
8. From the author's preface, Shaw GB: The Doctor's Dilemma. London, Constable, 1930, p xiii.
9. The argument is most explicitly stated and supported with empirical evidence in Monsma GN, Jr: Marginal revenue and the demand for physicians' services, in Klarman HE (ed): Empirical Studies in Health Economics: Proceedings of the Second Conference on the Economics of Health. Baltimore, The Johns Hopkins Press, 1970.
10. There is, in fact, persuasive evidence that the cost of health maintenance under prepayment plans is lower on a per capita basis than it is for the U.S. health care sector as a whole. Most of the savings appear to stem from lower utilization

of inpatient care. Indeed, the trade-off made by the prepaid plans between inpatient and outpatient care seems occasionally to increase the per capita utilization of ambulatory services. For an analysis of costs under prepayment and fee-for-service arrangements, see Anderson OW, Sheatsley PB: Comprehensive Medical Insurance: A Study of Costs, Use, and Attitudes Under Two Plans. Res Ser No. 9. New York, Health Information Foundation, 1959; National Advisory Commission on Health Manpower: Report, Vol. 1. Washington, D.C., U.S. Government Printing Office, 1967; Ellwood PM, Jr, O'Donoghue P, Hoagberg EJ, Schneider R, McClure W, Carlson RJ: Comparative analysis of a competitive HMO system with other health care delivery systems. Minneapolis, InterStudy, 1971 (mimeographed); and Roemer MI, Hetherington RW, Hopkins CE, Gerst AE, Parsons E, Long DM: Health Insurance Effects: Services, Expenditures, and Attitudes Under Three Types of Plan. Bur Public Health Econ Res Ser No. 16. Ann Arbor, School of Public Health, University of Michigan, 1972.

11. Pauly MV: Efficiency, incentives, and reimbursement for health care. Inquiry 7:114–131, 1970.
12. Freidson E: Professional Dominance: The Social Structure of Medical Care. New York, Atherton Press, 1970.
13. National Advisory Commission on Health Manpower: Report, Vol. 1. Washington, D.C., U.S. Government Printing Office, 1967; Newhouse JP: The economics of group practice. J Human Resour 8(1):37–56, 1973.
14. Donabedian A: An evaluation of prepaid group practice. Inquiry 6:3–27, 1969.
15. Klarman HE: Approaches to moderating the increases in medical care costs. Med Care 8(3):175–190 (May–June 1969).
16. Gonzales AF, Jr: West German medicine: Verrrry interesting. Prism 1:39–42, 1973.
17. Gerber A: Yes, there is a doctor shortage. Prism 1(5):13–15 (August 1972).
18. *Ibid.*, in which Gerber proposes no less than a doubling of existing medical school capacity.
19. Reinhardt UE: Physician Productivity and the "Physician Shortage" in the United States. Cambridge, Mass., Ballinger, 1974.
20. Sloan FA: Lifetime earnings and the physician's choice of specialty. Ind Labor Relat Rev 24:47–56, 1970.
21. A survey of alternative economic models of physician behavior and a description of the owner-operator model is in Reinhardt UE: Physician Productivity, *op. cit.* (ref 19).
22. Reinhardt UE: A production function for physicians' services. Rev Econ Stat 54:55–66, 1972; Smith KR, Miller M, Golladay FL: An analysis of the optimal use of inputs in the production of medical services. J Human Resour 7:208–225, 1972; Yankauer A, Connelly JP, Feldman JJ: Physician productivity in the delivery of ambulatory care: Some findings from a survey of pediatricians. Med Care 8(1):35–46 (Jan–Feb 1970).
23. Reinhardt UE: A production function, *op. cit.* (ref 22).
24. Hughes EFX, Fuchs VR, Jacoby JE: Surgical workloads in a community practice. Surgery 71:315–372, 1972.
25. The author is currently working with Kenneth R. Smith on a paper evaluating the implications of the SSA ruling on physician productivity.

26. Levy MJ Jr: Levy's Nine Laws of the Disillusionment of the True Liberal. University, Vol. 47 (Winter 1970–1971). Princeton University Press, Princeton, N.J.
27. In view of this, Corollary Two of Levy's Fourth Law seems applicable, but tact and innate timidity dissuade the author from presenting it here.
28. Quoted in Taylor MG: The Administration of Health Insurance in Canada. Toronto, Oxford University Press, 1956.

JONATHAN SPIVAK
Washington Bureau, The Wall Street Journal

Conference Commentary

In 1969, many experts assumed the time was ripe for adoption of national health insurance. Congress seemed prepared politically to launch the country in new directions in health care delivery and it was only up to the academics to tell the lawmakers what to do. Now five years later the blithe assumption that Congress is poised to pass sweeping new solutions to the problems of financing and delivering health services no longer appears valid.

The costs of government health programs like Medicaid and Medicare have skyrocketed and the problems of controlling hospital charges and physician fees have taken priority. Whatever new steps Congress chooses, its major concern will be assuring more effective regulation of the health industry.

The 1960s were a time of steady expansion of federal authority in the field of health care. Many precedents were shattered and most political barriers were broken. In a steady outpouring of legislation, Congress gave the federal government new responsibilities for treatment of mental health and mental retardation, expanded the infant and youth programs of the Children's Bureau, supported the construction of medical schools and the training of doctors, launched the Office of Economic Opportunity in its efforts to bring neighborhood health centers to the rural and urban ghettoes, and adopted the big federal financing programs—Medicare and Medicaid. In less than half a decade, Congress had moved the federal government from limited to massive involvement in the nation's medical care system. Washington was not only a major source of financial support for doctors, hospitals, and other providers of care but a decisive influence in the way health care was delivered.

But during these years of a rapid expansion, the bureaucrats' primary concern was to preserve the status quo and avoid controversy. Medicare adopted the conventional way of doing business by paying reasonable costs and its administrators at Social Security gave the private health industry a prime role in policymaking.

Only as health care costs escalated and the financial pressures mounted on federal budget makers did Washington begin to look askance at these arrangements. Increasingly, the politicians and the public demanded more forceful regulation and control. Federal health planners responded, but their solutions to the problem of cost control depended on their bias, legal authority, and willingness to take risks.

OEO and the Children's Bureau concentrated on comprehensive care and emphasized prevention; Medicaid tried to limit benefits and impose financial barriers on recipients; Medicare steadily tightened the screws in its reimbursement formula; the Public Health Service stressed regional planning efforts; and, superimposed on all these efforts, the Economic Stabilization Program sought to clamp a temporary national ceiling on medical care cost increases.

In a sense, this conference on regulation in the health industry has been a response to these historical developments. It has sought to determine if a consensus now exists on the best way to contain costs in the health industry. We have heard various arguments advanced: Some academics urge a return to the free market, while others advocate control by state health authorities, the widespread adoption of health maintenance organizations (HMOs), or incentive reimbursement arrangements. While no consensus has emerged, agreement appears to exist in some areas.

The first conclusion is that unfettered free enterprise cannot be relied on to control health care costs. Criticism by the opponents of strong federal regulation has emphasized that there is already too much governmental intervention in the medical marketplace. They point to the concentration of purchasing power in the Medicare program, the lack of incentives for efficiency inherent in cost-based reimbursement, and the consumer's lack of financial responsibility for his own care. All this unduly interferes with the free play of economic forces in the medical marketplace, they contend, and want to have unfettered supply and demand solve the problem. But their approach is impractical and unrealistic.

The political forces that propelled the government into the business of health care are far too powerful now to permit it to withdraw. Federal dollars make up nearly 40 percent of the health care pie and their influence cannot be avoided.

Sometimes the effects are unintended. The sudden and vast expansion of federal–state Medicaid programs was completely unanticipated when the legislation was adopted by Congress in 1965. At other times federal financing brings surprisingly little change. Medicare money failed to stimulate growth of community-based home health care organizations, although these arrangements were obviously desirable for the program and for patients.

Whatever the outcome, the fiscal ties between federal programs and health care institutions are now so strong that it is silly to think of severing them. Nonregulation in the health care field is an interesting academic concept, but not a viable alternative.

If regulation is inevitable, what should its objective be? There appears little doubt from the concerns expressed at this conference that the awesome expense of medical treatment is the issue that grips the politicians and the public. That is the problem that regulators, whether in Washington or in state government, will have to deal with, and *not* arguable reforms in the delivery of health care.

In the late 1960s, Johnson administration budget men were becoming alarmed at the inflationary increases in health care costs that followed the adoption of Medicare and Medicaid. Later, the Nixon administration also agonized over control of rising health costs. Mr. Nixon's first HEW secretary, Robert Finch, sounded the strategic concern in a 1971 white paper on the "crisis in health care." The two primary problems were inflation's impact on existing health care programs and the demand for new benefits to relieve the financial pressure on consumers.

Between 1967 and 1973, total public and private spending for health care rose from $47.9 billion, or 6.2 percent of the Gross National Product, to $94.1 billion, or 7.7 percent of GNP. The conference experts appeared to agree that medical outlays will not continue indefinitely to absorb a greater share of GNP. The primary political objective will be to fashion a rational system of regulation that will moderate cost increases and make medical outlays more predictable for government and consumer.

But the agreement ends there. Although the quality and quantity of basic data have vastly improved over the years, its interpretation still remains subject to dispute. Some people say that HMOs have reduced hospitalization by putting the financial incentives on preventive care and outpatient treatment. Others argue that the savings result from undue restrictions and often conceal the fact that HMO patients seek hospital care outside the program.

There is conflict over standards and objectives. We do not know how to measure health. Can we rely on mortality rate to indicate the effectiveness of a nation's health care system, or are there better indices? Is it important that people think they are better, and if so how do we make such subjective measurements?

In some ways the health debate now taking place resembles the one that rent the field of public education a few years back. Educators tried to determine if federal programs actually improved the schools, but no one could agree on the measures to use. Many of the conferees here and in other health care debates are themselves providers of care or services. Hospitals, physicians, and private insurers can hardly be unbiased when their economic well-being is involved. Even the academics have their professional prestige at stake. While the health industry is dominated by "nonprofit" institutions, their growth and influence are dependent on the same financial factors that affect money-making organizations.

Has a convincing case been made at this conference for any one scheme of cost control? The answer is no. Some experts argue that quality of service is the important issue, not cost. But confusion over measurement methods makes this approach questionable. Most would agree it is easier to let the new Professional Standards Review Organizations grapple with this problem.

Others argue that limits might be imposed on the frequency of care, but this is difficult as a practical matter. Once a benefit is established in law and public funds are furnished, demands become rights. There is no equitable way to limit the availability of care. The costly chronic kidney disease benefit under Medicare shows that politically vulnerable government administrators cannot pick and choose patients, even though doctors might have valid medical reasons to do so.

Some have suggested that regulation focus on the professionals who deliver health care. Physicians could be forced into under-manned specialties or told where to practice so as to insure that the supply is adequate and demand does not drive up prices.

The enthusiasm here for this approach seems surprising. Setting quotas for specialists and dispatching physicians to the rural hinterlands represent radical departures from past practice. The government has not chosen to impose such restraints on other professional groups and, besides, health experts cannot agree on desired physician–population ratios.

We are back then to cost controls as the only politically feasible approach—one that appeals as much to liberals as conservatives. But each alternative method has disadvantages.

Health Maintenance Organizations The definition of *HMO* remains debatable and, without agreement on its precise characteristics, assessment is impossible. We do not know whether HMOs will save money, improve or debase the quality of care, remain static or spread. This conference shows that, if anything, the controversy over HMOs will continue for some time.

Certification of Need Geographical franchising of hospital beds has also failed to control rising hospital costs. Indeed, the major problem now appears to be eliminating unused bed capacity (which franchising will not remedy), rather than preventing new beds (which it will).

State Rate Control Only a handful of states have moved in this direction and it is far too early to determine their impact. Extensive efforts by Maryland are not due to be fully in effect until mid-1974. And we will be arguing over the value of state regulation for many more months.

Economic Stabilization Controls The government's new approach to rate regulation, which is being tested in the courts, promises to be simpler and more effective than past efforts. But hospital administrators question whether they have sufficient authority over physicians, the men whose decisions really count, to abide by any government-imposed limitation on costs.

Medicare and Medicaid Controls Washington bureaucrats run programs that pay for more than a third of the hospital care in the country, but their cost-control efforts have not been impressive. In Medicaid, power is diffuse and HEW officials must cajole and persuade state counterparts to implement their decisions. The Social Security Administration has a far more centralized authority in Medicare, but is reluctant to exert its influence or threaten the providers.

If none of the approaches discussed at this conference appears to work, where do we go from here? The major target of opportunity remains the hospital. And while most administrators concede there is little prospect of preventing cost increases, the rise can be slowed.

Under any new national health insurance program Congress appears likely to cover the cost of catastrophic illness for the middle class and lift the mounting fiscal burden of Medicaid from the states. The challenge facing medical experts and consumers of health care is to capitalize on these political pressures by imposing better methods of cost control on the health industry.

And since the experts often cannot agree on how to do it, the most essential task will be to devise ways by which the ideas of health care consumers can be introduced into the debate and adopted.

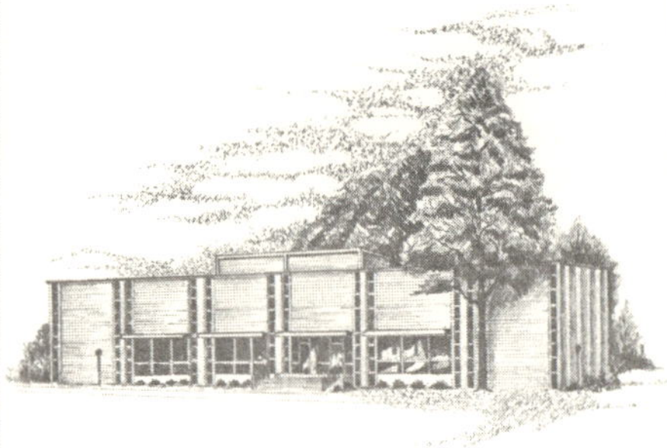